WARREN COLE, MD, AND THE ASCENT OF SCIENTIFIC SURGERY

Dennis Connaughton

The Warren and Clara Cole Foundation, Publishers
Chicago

Distributed by the University of Illinois Press
Champaign, Ill.

For information about this book, address The Warren and Clara Cole Foundation, 55 East Erie Street, Chicago, IL 60611.

Library of Congress Catalog Card Number 91-65-266

Printed in the United States of America

ISBN 0-9628799-0-8

Book designed by Jean Farley Brown

Dust jacket designed by Fred Semmler

Sketch of Dr. Cole on dust jacket was adapted from a drawing by Danforth Robinson that appeared in *Imago Chirugii*, published by Ethicon Inc., Somerville, N.J.

Composition by Norman Wald

Contents

PREFACE

Academic professors in medical school are generally measured by their achievements in teaching, research and clinical practice, the classical three-legged stool to which an administrative leg may be grudgingly added. Current emphasis on the economics of health care, especially the continuing need for medical centers to extract large sums from full-time surgical practices, has tended to relegate research and teaching to lesser roles in the academic hierarchy.

For the young men and women in medical school and residency, however, teaching is preeminently important, and Warren Cole was a brilliant exemplification of that principle. As a surgical professor whose life spanned the better part of a century, one-third of it as a departmental chairman, we might expect a large cadre of students and associates whose careers were significantly affected by his teaching.

But the intensity of affectionate loyalty that he generated among his disciples far exceeded the conventional master and pupil relationship. For example, during the decade before his death, large numbers of former residents and their spouses traveled annually to his retirement home in Asheville to celebrate his birthday.

Dennis Connaughton was able to meet with Doctor and Mrs. Cole in the course of winnowing through the ample professional and personal records of this quiet, undemonstrative man. He has captured nicely the reasons for Warren Cole's significant influence for a quarter century after he retired from a prestigious university chairmanship in surgery. During that period of normal retirement, he wrote three books and 24 articles, almost exclusively as sole author.

Best known for his pioneer work with Evarts Graham on cholecystography, Doctor Cole made fundamental contributions as well to the management of cancer and to many other surgical problems. An honorary member of more than 20 national and international societies, he achieved presidential office in most of the great surgical organizations and was the recipient of civic honors in full measure.

Despite all this, he maintained the unaffected simplicity that the author has captured in this splendid account of a country boy whose mother's death after a kitchen-table hysterectomy triggered his resolve to improve the quality of surgical practice. How well he succeeded in his lifelong quest is strikingly portrayed in this inspiring story of Warren Cole's role in the rise of scientific surgery during most of this century.

His selfless spirit lives on in the educational foundation that he and Mrs. Cole endowed in the last years of his life, and in the Warren H. Cole Society that honors and perpetuates the memory of this stalwart crusader for better surgical care.

C. Rollins Hanlon, MD
President of The Warren and Clara Cole Foundation

INTRODUCTION

࿉

Shortly after Dr. C. Rollins Hanlon first contacted me in the spring of 1989 about writing this biography, I received three large cardboard boxes filled with the private papers of Dr. Warren H. Cole.

At the time, I knew of Dr. Cole only as a former president of the American College of Surgeons. For 11 years, from 1977 to 1988, I had been editor of a monthly magazine published by the College, the *Bulletin of the American College of Surgeons*. Dr. Cole was still alive then, but I never had the opportunity to meet him.

And so I began plowing through those three cardboard cartons with very little background to the man and his work. The boxes contained, among other things, private letters dating from the 1930s to the 1980s, confidential reports, and reminiscences of his life written in his retirement years.

There were also transcripts of a taped interview with Dr. Cole conducted by Dr. G. Howard Glassford, one of Cole's former residents, who had done the interview as a prelude to writing the Cole biography himself. But surgery is a demanding profession, and Dr. Glassford never got beyond the backgrounding stage. Those interviews were invaluable to me, however, because they gave me my first personal glimpse into the man represented by the papers before me.

The more I read of Dr. Cole's papers, the more I was struck by the fact that his life represented not only the saga of a man of medicine but also the story of the development of surgery in the 20th century. It was medical history as seen through the eyes of one man who contributed significantly to its evolution. And so that was the approach I took to writing his biography.

In December of same year, 1989, I flew to Asheville, North Carolina, where Dr. Cole was living in retirement, to interview him for this book. It was a scant six months before his death. He was 91 years old. He was at the time living in a retirement community called Givens Estates with his wife Clara. I remember him greeting me at the front door to the building in which they lived with great zest and energy.

He was a thin, strong man who looked younger than his 91 years and whose mind was as sharp as most people half his age. That evening and throughout the next day, he recounted for me some major events in his life with the precision of a research scientist and the affection of a man who seemed eminently fulfilled.

I will not easily forget the clarity of his memories of his mother's kitchen-table operation, an incident that took place 85 years previously, yet was recreated for me in vivid detail. He was a master storyteller and he relished bringing his memories to life.

For months after that visit, Dr. Cole would call me in Chicago to give me some information he thought I could use or to clarify something he had told me when I visited Asheville. He wanted to make sure that whatever I wrote about him was true, accurate and not overstated. That was the way he conducted his life.

Many people had a hand in developing this book, and I need to acknowledge some of them. First are the members of the Warren Cole Society who promoted the idea of writing Dr. Cole's biography and who helped finance the project. Next is Dr. Hanlon, president of The Warren and Clara Cole Foundation, who was my guide and mentor from beginning to end. He allowed and encouraged me to expand the scope of the book beyond a narrow biography to include the history of surgery and medical education.

My thanks go to Robert Adelsperger and Sandra Young at the University of Illinois Health Sciences Library in Chicago, who gave me access to the library's special collections, and to William Maher at the University of Illinois Library in Urbana, who opened the archives to me. Also thanks to Cecile Kramer, director of the medical library at Northwestern University Medical School in Chicago, and to Marjorie Williams, who edited the book with a deft touch.

SECTION ONE:

THE KANSAS YEARS

CHAPTER 1

❧

SURGERY ON THE KITCHEN TABLE

The surgeon came by horse and buggy, moving quickly through the Kansas countryside to reach his patient before she bled to death. Summoned by a rural physician to perform a hysterectomy on a woman who had developed persistent vaginal bleeding after a miscarriage, the surgeon was traveling from Topeka to a farm about six miles northwest of Clay Center, Kansas, a distance of about 85 miles. The year was 1904. The woman was Sophia Tolin Cole, the mother of Warren Cole, who was then five years old. The operation would be performed in the kitchen of the family's farmhouse.

Kitchen-table operations by itinerant surgeons were still common in rural areas around the turn of the century. There was no hospital in Clay Center, a town of a few thousand people located near the Republican River in east-central Kansas.

Even if there had been, the general fear of hospitals at that time was still so great that many people avoided them at all costs, and for good reason. Operative mortality rates were high—some claim because patients resisted advice to go to a hospital and delayed their operations too long—and infections swept through hospitals, sometimes in epidemic proportions, resulting in deaths from causes unrelated to the reason the patient entered the hospital. Cross-infection from one patient to another could result in fatal bouts of hospital gangrene, erysipelas (an inflammatory disease caused by a streptococcus) and pyemia—poisoning of the blood by microorganisms.

When the surgeon arrived, the children—five boys, of whom Warren was the next to youngest—were led out of the house into the late-spring day. After he examined Warren's mother, the surgeon confirmed the local doctor's diagnosis and prepared to operate. Years later, Warren's father, George Cole, told him that a family member had overheard the nurse who was present to assist the surgeon say, "But Doctor, you can't operate on her. She is too anemic. She will die." Her warning went unheeded.

The Cole family had made preparations for the operation while the surgeon was en route. They selected the kitchen because it was well lighted. After they removed all the furniture and wall hangings from the room, they scrubbed the floor and walls and nailed sheets to the windows to keep the children and neighbors from peering in during the operation. The day before the operation, one of the family members filled a wash boiler halfway with water, boiled it on the stove for an hour or so and allowed it to cool overnight. A teakettle or two of water was also boiled and cooled.

After the surgeon arrived, the kitchen table was covered with a sheet, and a kitchen chair was set beside it to be used as an instrument table. The surgical instruments were boiled in the family dishpan. Kerosene lamps were lit to provide extra illumination. It was typical of the time that if sterilized gauze was not available, towels were cut up to be used as sponges and boiled with the instruments. In addition, a whole towel would be boiled and then placed around the site of the operation. When necessary, the patient's body hair was shaved if a razor was available; if the family had no razor, which was sometimes the case because of the popularity of whiskers, the hair was clipped with a pair of scissors and the stubble scrubbed with homemade lye soap.

Although primitive by today's standards, Sophia Cole's operation was fairly typical of what medical science had to offer at the time. Rubber surgical gloves had become available just before the turn of the century, but many surgeons at first resisted their use, insisting that they reduced the sensitivity of touch. Instead, they washed their hands thoroughly with soap and scrubbed under their fingernails with brushes. Sophia's surgeon and his assistant would have worn white surgical gowns at that time, but not masks and caps. Some of Sophia's clothes would have been left on for protection; clothing was usually cleaner than the available bed covering, and many households had only feather comforters on the beds.

Strict adherence to cleanliness or aseptic practice was an outgrowth of the germ theory of disease—that bacteria spread infection—and a natural progression in medicine from the antiseptic techniques promoted by the great English surgeon Joseph Lister. Basing his theses on the research done by Louis Pasteur on putrefaction and the contamination of sterile fluids, Lister first began in 1865 to apply carbolic acid to wounds to kill germs, and later, in 1871, he began to spray the air in operating rooms with carbolic acid spray on the theory that the air was a significant source of infection.

By 1880, most doctors began to accept Lister's germicidal techniques without actually having heard of the germ theory itself. Lister's work brought successful results, and it was practical and easy to repeat. The germ theory revolutionized medicine from ritualism to scientific practice and set the stage for modern surgery. Between 1880 and 1900, in rapid-fire succession, the bacteria responsible for dozens of diseases were discovered. From Germany came news of Robert Koch's discovery of the bacterium responsible for tuberculosis in 1882, and the cholera bacillus the next year. In 1884, Klebs and Loeffler announced the discovery of the diphtheria bacillus, and in 1893, Emil Behring demonstrated successful treatment of diphtheria with diphtheria antiserum. In 1894, Shibasabura Kitasato and Alexandre Yersin independently discovered the germ that had caused bubonic plague. These and other discoveries opened up a new world of protection against disease through immunization.

It was Koch who pointed out that most antiseptics fail to destroy bacteria but merely retard the growth of organisms. In 1881, he showed that heat was superior to chemicals in destroying and inhibiting bacterial action. He then invented a process of sterilization by steam. Despite debates back and forth about the validity of the germ theory, surgeons in the 1880s gradually began to realize that clothes, instruments, sheets and their own hands rather than the air of the operating room were the sources of disease-bearing germs. Soap, sterilization and rigid rules of cleanliness replaced sprays and harsh germicides for operations. Surgical gowns had replaced frock coats and aprons caked with blood and pus.

Another revolution that occurred in the 19th century and was to have a profound effect on medicine in general and the practice of surgery in particular was the discovery of anesthetics. Before the second half of the 19th century, people were so terrified of surgery that they would refuse or delay operations if at all possible; in some cases, for example, patients would allow tumors to grow to 50 or 100 pounds before having them removed. Various substances were used to reduce pain, including opium, hemp, hashish and whiskey, but a safe and sure anesthetic that would affect all patients in the same way was lacking. It wasn't until the early 1840s that nitrous oxide, or laughing gas, came into vogue, even though the gas itself had been discovered in 1772 by Joseph Priestley. In 1844, a Hartford dentist named Horace Wells saw a fairground demonstration of laughing gas and noted that a volunteer was unaware of a severe cut he sustained in his knee during the demonstration.

Another dentist, Bostonian William Morton, is credited, along with his partner Charles Jackson, with developing ether as an anesthetic. In 1845, Morton saw Wells demonstrate the use of nitrous oxide for pain-free tooth extraction, a demonstration that failed, and thought of ether as an alternative. Morton suggested to Harvard surgeon John Collins Warren that ether could be useful in surgery. (A surgeon in Georgia, Crawford W. Long, had been using ether successfully for operations since 1842, but he had not published his results.) In 1846, the day after Warren first used it during an operation to remove a tumor from a patient's neck, the Boston papers headlined the story. Within a short time, ether was being used in operating rooms across the United States.

While ether was a uniquely American contribution to the advancement of surgery, the use of chloroform, the other major anesthetic in use at the time of Sophie Cole's operation, resulted from a Scottish obstetrician's dissatisfaction with ether. At the suggestion of a chemist in Liverpool, James Y. Simpson began to experiment with chloroform in Edinburgh, and, in 1847, began to use it to ease the pain of childbirth for his patients. When Queen Victoria accepted it for the birth of her eighth child, chloroform became all the rage.

While anesthesia in the form of ether or chloroform was available at the time of Sophie Cole's operation, as late as 1895 anesthetics were used in Kansas only for hospital surgery. Many deaths had occurred when inexperienced students or nurses administered the substances, which were not yet well understood. Most country surgeons there continued to rely on whiskey to alleviate pain when operations were done in the home. It is very likely, however, that by 1904 the surgeon from Topeka would have administered chloroform or ether.

In a popular book written in 1938, *Horse and Buggy Doctor*, surgeon Arthur E. Hertzler, a world authority on local anesthesia, described what it was like to do kitchen surgery at the turn of the century in the central Kansas town of Halstead, where he practiced. "Those doctors who were trained in the Southern medical schools," he wrote, "preferred to use chloroform and usually gave it with a high degree of skill, but I was always frightened when it was being used. I saw one fine young schoolteacher die from degeneration of the liver following chloroform anesthesia. After this, I refused to permit its use. This girl haunts me still. Chloroform had another distinct disadvantage at night. This drug, when the vapors are exposed to the flame of the kerosene lamp, disintegrates and produces a terribly irritating gas. I once battled with a perforated ulcer of the duodenum under these conditions for an hour and it was only by the exercise of all the will power I possessed that I was able to finish the operation, because of the irritation produced in my bronchial tubes by this gas."

Ether was usually unskillfully given, Hertzler noted, and it usually took an hour or more to get the patient asleep.

In wide use at the time was the drop method, by which the anesthetist—usually the local doctor or nurse—slowly dripped ether from a vial onto a cloth covering the patient's mouth and nose.

"All that is necessary in the performance of an aseptic operation," commented Hertzler, "is a reasonably clean skin—for no matter how elaborate the preparation, it is not really clean, only reasonably clean—a few clean tools and, of course, an operator who knows what it is all about."

Surgeons used silk for sutures at the time, and Mrs. Cole's surgeon surely would have tied off the blood vessels before he cut them. However, suturing of vessels was being done only on an experimental basis. Speed was a vital factor in kitchen-table operations, on the theory that the more quickly the operation was performed, the less trauma there would be to tissue.

Following the operation came the problems of dressing and aftercare. Obviously, elaborate postoperative care was not available, and for the most part, itinerant surgeons dressed the wound after the operation and left the patient alone to heal. "In dressing the wound after operation, one had to evaluate the intelligence of those who were to care for the patient after the surgeon left," wrote Hertzler. "The most explicit instructions to leave the dressings undisturbed had little effect on many of the old doctors. In a few days after the operation, when the patient was fever-free, the delighted doctor would become curious to see what made the patient do so well and he would remove the dressings. These doctors usually dated back to the days of 'laudable pus' when every well-behaved wound was supposed to suppurate. In several instances the patient complained of pain from the sutures, usually in twelve or twenty-four hours after the operation, and the doctor would obligingly remove them."

Medical education before the turn of the century was hampered by shoddy commercialism and low standards. It was possible for someone to get a medical degree from a correspondence school or "read medicine" with an older practitioner and then go into practice. Proprietary medical schools, unaffiliated with a university, sprang up across the nation in the 19th century, and in their greed to attract students and make money, they competed with one another by shortening the curriculum and easing the requirements for degrees. An outgrowth of the rampant spirit of free enterprise and laissez-faire that was characteristic of this era in American history, the schools were owned and operated by the faculty and depended on student fees for income. They were businesses rather than educational institutions, and they measured their success by the numbers they graduated and the profits they made.

The standard curriculum consisted of seven courses: anatomy; physiology and pathology; materia medica, therapeutics and pharmacy; chemistry and medical jurisprudence; theory and practice of medicine; principles and practice of surgery; and obstetrics and diseases of women and children. The courses were taught in lectures given over two terms lasting four months each during winter; the second term was a repeat of the first. Most students graduated with skills that were hopelessly deficient.

Some organizers tried to set up proprietary medical colleges all over Kansas as well, although few got beyond the charter stage. The schools required virtually no preliminary education of their students and hired so-called professors from the ranks of the local medical profession. One of the more successful proprietary schools of this era, the Kansas Medical College, which was founded in Topeka in 1890, created a scandal when the city's newspaper, the *Topeka Capital*, revealed that the school was solving its lack of sufficient anatomical material for dissections by robbing the graves of a local cemetery.

Standards were so low in American medical schools that anyone serious about a good medical education went to Europe for postgraduate training. Americans flocked to Europe, but Europeans shunned American schools. In the first half of the 19th century, France was the students' mecca; after 1850, Germany replaced France as their first choice. The revolution toward scientific medicine had begun in Europe long before it got under way in America, but the European influence set the forces for reform in motion in the United States toward the end of the 19th century, and its momentum redefined medical education in the early 20th century.

All of these factors of medical knowledge and education came to bear on the operation performed on Warren Cole's mother. A seminal event in Dr. Cole's life, the operation is one of his earliest memories.

In December of 1989, when he was 91 years old, Dr. Cole remembered that after the operation was completed, he and his four brothers were brought into the kitchen to gather around their mother. He recalled his mother lying on the table, the kerosene lamps glowing and the surgeon in a white gown. "My father was pretty upset, naturally," he said. "They must have told me she was dying, but I didn't know what that meant. I felt a strange sense that something catastrophic had happened, although I didn't know what it was. I tried to look around at the people present. There were quite a few. My mother had several sisters, and I presume they were all there. It made me think that something important was happening, but I wasn't quite able to understand what it was."

A few days after the operation was performed, on May 18, 1904, Sophia Cole died. She was 31 years old. Her death certificate did not list the cause of death.

According to Dr. Cole, Sophie came from a large family in Clay Center. Her father was a farmer who was well known and liked in town, and Warren described Sophia's mother as matriarchal. Sophie Tolin married George Cole in 1888 when she was 15 years old. Together they forged a farm from the wilderness and produced five boys: Perry, Cecil, Irvin, Warren and Louis. Her death made Warren's father so bitter about the medical profession that he almost prevented Warren from becoming a doctor in later years.

In 1986, while in retirement in Asheville, North Carolina, Dr. Cole wrote: "Naturally, I must have missed my mother very much at the time, but I recall so little about my mother that I have only a faint recollection of her appearance and her actions. I have often heard people use the loss of a mother in early childhood as an excuse for their failure— whether it be misbehavior, lack of intelligence, inability to concentrate, etc. I realize a mother's love is very precious but I refuse to condone the failures of children, especially a boy, on her loss. I choose to blame my deficiencies on myself, not on the loss of my mother. This is, of course, assuming that the child has a father or someone to guide and counsel him."

If anything, Sophie Cole's death after a kitchen-table operation was a spur to Warren to devote his life to surgery; he wanted to improve the lot of the surgical patient and help prevent death from operations. By the time he retired from his position as chairman of the department of surgery at the University of Illinois in 1966, he had made major contributions to the fields of surgery and radiology. His work with such organizations as the American College of Surgeons and the American Cancer Society—he became president of both groups—helped eliminate the primitive conditions under which his mother was operated on and died.

At the time of Warren Cole's birth on July 24, 1898, surgery was rapidly developing from a crude and dangerous art to an influential medical specialty based on scientific research and discovery. The advent of anesthetics and the means to prevent wound infection during the 19th century laid the groundwork for a century of unprecedented advancement in man's war against the ravages of disease. From the earliest days of recorded history until the 19th century, surgery had offered little in curing disease and had improved almost not at all. Over the past century, modern miracles have been achieved in organ transplantations, cancer surgery and immunotherapy, vastly improved operating techniques, far superior training of surgical interns and residents, and virtually every aspect of surgical practice.

Warren Cole's contributions to the advancement of medical science and the teaching of surgery are legion. He was a man who came into history at the right time with an inquisitive mind capable of helping to unravel some of the mysteries of modern medicine. He and Dr. Evarts Graham made an original and lasting contribution to the detection of gallbladder disease and the entire field of diagnostic radiology with their discovery of cholecystography. He made a major contribution to the battle against cancer with a description of how cancer cells shed into the blood stream. And he devoted his career to improving surgical education as department chairman at the University of Illinois.

As an indication of his standing in the history of medicine in the 20th century, Dr. Cole was honored by the scientific and academic medical community in various ways. A member of 31 medical and scientific societies, he became president of 15 of these organizations. He received some 23 honors and awards and was made an honorary member of 22 medical societies. He was a visiting professor at major universities 17 times and served on the editorial boards of eight scientific journals.

Dr. Cole's life story is the story of the growth of scientific medicine and the work of one of the great innovators in surgical science and education.

CHAPTER 2

❧

LIFE ON THE FARM

One day before Warren Cole was born on July 24, 1898, according to records filed with the Clay County Register of Deeds, Warren's father George and his uncle Eli, George's brother, purchased the last parcel of land, some 160 acres at a price of $5,000, that made up their jointly held farmlands in Clay County, Kansas.

George Cole was born in Lancaster, Pennsylvania in 1856. A few years later, just as the rumblings of Civil War were threatening to rend the fabric of the Union, the Cole family moved to a farm in Waterloo, Illinois, a town about 15 miles southeast of St. Louis. Waterloo was just north of Bellefontaine, the first English-speaking settlement in Illinois, which was established in 1779 and noted for the richness of its soil. As English-speaking settlers gradually filled the area, the entire region became known as the American Bottom to help distinguish it from the Spanish territory on the west bank of the Mississippi.

Although the beginning of the Civil War in 1861 created a deep depression for the farmers of the North because the corn, wheat, barreled pork and whiskey normally sold in the South began to pile up in warehouses, supplying the needs of the Union army and three years of bad weather and crop failures in Europe soon triggered an economic recovery. Chicago became a major trading center and that fact, along with the growth of railroads, spelled a boon for Illinois farmers throughout the war and in the years beyond.

Southern Illinois, however, had the disadvantage of being bordered by two slave states—Missouri and Kentucky— and as a result, it was the scene of frequent skirmishes between sympathizers of one side or the other. The farmers of the area found themselves caught in the middle. Young George Cole grew up in this environment, and evidently the hostility surrounding him made him long for serener pastures.

His son Warren described the circumstances in this way: "The Civil War started when he was just a young boy. However, we were never able to get him to talk much about the Civil War. One of the reasons may have been his young age, but I suspect the dangerous features of living in Southern Illinois on the line between the North and the South led to many disagreeable incidents which he did not wish to talk about. He worked on the farm for a few years, saving his money so he could go farther west and buy land somewhere in Kansas. Part of this trip was made by covered wagon."

In those days, Kansas was still the frontier. The great cattle drives north from Texas reached their peak in the late 1870s, and in the western part of the state, wild and woolly Dodge City, as the citizens of eastern Kansas called it, became Queen of the Cow Towns and home to such infamous gunslingers as Bat Masterson, Wyatt Earp and Doc Holliday, the town's first dentist. In the 1880s, encouraged by favorable weather conditions and glowing reports of high crop yields, immigrants flooded into Kansas at record rates. Census figures show that between 1880 and 1890, the number of Kansas residents jumped by nearly 50 percent to more than 1.4 million, the biggest increase in the state's history.

Many came up the Missouri by steamboat from St. Louis to Kansas City, then finished their trek in covered wagons. George Cole and his two brothers, John and Eli, arrived in Clay Center by covered wagon in 1881. On April 5, they purchased 80 acres of farmland six miles northwest of town for $1,000. A year later, on September 9, the three brothers bought another 160 acres of adjoining land for $4,000. In

1884, John Cole sold his interest in the land to his brothers for $3,000 and apparently moved to Nebraska. The next year, George and Eli bought about 68 acres of fertile land along the Republican River for $1,600, and in 1892 and 1893, the two brothers deeded land to one another so that each held title to separate farms. By the time Warren Cole was born, his father owned about 255 acres of farmland.

George Cole built a two-story frame house on the land and, in 1885, planted a cottonwood tree in front of the house that grew nearly four stories tall and survived well into the next century. He married Sophia Tolin, a 15-year-old girl from a local farm, in 1888, when he was 32, and began raising boys as well as wheat.

Dr. Cole remembered his father as "a quiet individual who had no obvious temper. He was someone who devoted his life to providing the necessities for the family. I liked my father very much. He was always good to us, yet he carried, shall we say, a club in case there were any arguments. He would settle them. He was a very thoughtful individual and loved the family."

After Sophia died, George advertised for a housekeeper in the two Kansas City newspapers that he read avidly. "We must have had eight or ten housekeepers during the period following my mother's death until my father remarried at the time I graduated from high school," Dr. Cole remembered. "He was able to judge their character from the applicants' letters in answer to the ads; seldom did we get a dud. With few exceptions, these housekeepers were splendid individuals who were willing to work hard and were very considerate of our family.

"Nevertheless, father would make no effort to replace help during the winter months since demands in the fields were practically nil, which allowed us boys plenty of time to attend to household chores.

"When I was seven or eight years old, strange as it seems," Dr. Cole said in 1989, "I fell heir to the cooking responsibility when the housekeeper was not there. Apparently I was able to do it without much trouble. I cooked potatoes and rice and other things that were easily cooked. Of course, we also had a lot of help from our aunts and neighbors."

About 120 acres of George Cole's farm were devoted to growing wheat, another 100 acres were planted with corn, 25 acres were filled with alfalfa, and timothy hay took up the remaining 10 acres, which consisted of sand knolls that were not tilled because of the threat of drifting sand.

The early settlers of Kansas had come from the corn states to the east and naturally planted corn on their new farms. But the early 1870s brought depression, grasshoppers and drought, and in 1874, the corn crop was severely damaged and in some places destroyed. Also injured were spring wheat and other small grains, and so the farmers turned to winter wheat. By 1875, the State Board of Agriculture was convinced that wheat, especially winter wheat, was a safer crop than corn and sold the idea to farmers. Its annual report of that year warned Kansans: "Don't put all your eggs in the corn basket; put most in the wheat basket, it is safer."

Wheat production depended on labor-saving devices, such as harvesters, threshing machines and windmills. Railroads were necessary to carry the grain to market, and fences and herd laws protected the crops from roaming cattle. All of these developments were established by the time George Cole started his farm.

"I consider myself extremely fortunate to have been born and raised on the farm," Dr. Warren Cole wrote in his retirement years. "There are numerous advantages in this life which cannot be equalled by living in the city. Life on a farm and going to a country school were, in my estimation, very advantageous to my future, largely because of the many character-building hardships we had to undergo. In my opinion, these hardships develop character, that is, tolerance, patience, willingness to work hard and many other desirable characteristics. This is not to say that I have these qualities, but I am saying that I was not a spoiled brat, which is the kind of character some youngsters develop who live in the city and have all the material things they want."

During the summertime, farm hands were hired to harvest the wheat, but George and his five boys did most of the other work on the farm. "When I was a youngster," Warren Cole wrote in 1981, "the greatest day of the year was when the steam engines pulled the thresher into my dad's fields and started threshing the wheat." The thresher, which was run by a steam engine with a series of belts that rotated wheels, separated the grain from the wheat plant. Farmers pitched wheat into the thresher from the sides, and one man stood on top to watch the operation and make sure all the mechanisms were functioning properly.

Winter wheat was planted in the fall, while corn was planted in April and had to be cultivated as the wheat was growing. "Shortly after the corn came up," Dr. Cole wrote, "we went over it with a weed cutter equipped with a huge knife blade on each side that cut into the dirt wall made by the lister when the corn was planted. The weed cutter not only got rid of the weeds but leveled the ground as well. The corn had to be cultivated at least twice during the growing season. Although outside farm hands were needed to perform odd jobs, such as cutting and putting up hay, my brothers and I did most of the work on the farm and had plenty to do during the spring and summer months. My younger brother, Louis, was too small to qualify as a farm hand. Although I did most of the cooking, I was still required to take a team and help with the cultivating or attend to some other needed chore.

"Harvest time is the most important in a farmer's life. Even with us boys on the farm, my father needed to hire help at threshing time. My brother Irvin, who had a mechanical bent—he later studied agriculture at Kansas State in Manhattan, Kansas—ran the binder when the wheat ripened. About two weeks were spent in cutting the wheat, but the biggest and hardest task was shocking the wheat. The wheat bundles, after binding, had to be put up in shocks to avoid being ruined by dampness on the ground, not to mention rain and hail. Inevitably, it fell to my lot to help with the shocking, since at least three men were needed to keep up with the binder. I can still remember the tiresome task—the endless process of walking to the next bundle, picking it up and returning it to the shock. What fatigue! Under the blazing sun, day after day, it seemed interminable. The discipline needed to perform such work surely built character. During these times, father always saw to it that we had a housekeeper so that all the boys could concentrate on field work.

We accomplished most of the work of harvesting the wheat, corn and alfalfa (which had to be cut four times a year starting in early May).

"About the time I started high school [1910], the automatic wheat cutter and thresher combine came into use. The farmers were somewhat reluctant to use this machine, partly because cutting had to be delayed a week beyond binding time before the wheat could be threshed with the combine. Furthermore, the machine was extremely costly—$4,000 to $5,000—at a time when very few farmers could afford it.

"During my years on the farm, we had threshing machines that consisted of a steam engine and a thresher, called a separator. This was usually an exciting time for us youngsters and for father, too, because of the tremendous responsibility it represented. The farmers cooperated fully with each other in performing this work. Threshing required six men and teams of horses pulling a hayrack and four to eight wagons to carry the wheat to the granary or to town.

"When I was too small to run a hayrack, I was put to work hauling grain. Because the price of wheat was low at harvest time, my father and one of his close friends, a man I knew as Mr. Boge, scooped the wheat into the granary themselves to make sure none was lost. What a back-breaking job that was: the two men scooping wheat continuously all day long. I marvel at the endurance displayed by both my father and Mr. Boge, with neither suffering any back trouble. My father was not a large man, but he was very wiry and tough; his friend was a husky, strong individual. Because of our changes in habit today, I'm afraid the number of slipped discs from this kind of labor would be enormous.

"Perhaps the only job as strenuous as scooping wheat was the job that belonged to the so-called pitcher, who worked out in the wheat fields lifting bundles of wheat from the shock onto the hayrack. The pitcher was paid what was in those days a very high salary—one dollar a day. On hot days, and it seemed like all of them were hot, this task probably took more stamina than scooping wheat; the pitcher had to work in the sun while the scooper could work in the shade of the granary. It required four pitchers to keep the hayrack full of bundles to carry to the thresher.

"When I was too young to do any manual work, I found great pleasure in wandering around the fields and watching the engineer run his steam engine while the tender kept an eye on the separator—like a hawk watches his prey. The tender seemed to be running all day long from bearing to bearing with an oil can in hand in order to keep the complicated machinery going, all the while trying to shield the dust spewing from the threshing machine from his eyes, even though he wore goggles and a cap that overlapped his face.

"I considered running the hayrack to be the plum of all the threshing jobs. The pitcher would throw bundles of wheat into the hayrack; when the rack was full, farm hands would toss the bundles head first into the open mouth of the thresher, which was equipped with revolving knives that cut the binding twine and the wheat stalks. As the racks were emptied, more bundles were collected from the fields, and the work continued. Six or seven farmers cooperated with one another in this work; when all the wheat was threshed on one farm, the same crew moved on to the next.

"The threshing operation required a lot of consultation time between neighboring farmers; this was made possible by the introduction of the telephone into rural areas, something that took place only two or three years before I was born. The telephone brought a remarkable era to farm life, when one individual could listen to the conversations of neighbors—what a great privilege that was!

"Shortly after threshing was completed, plowing—an exhausting and monotonous job—began. Each plow required three horses to pull it and could plow under only an acre and a half in one day. A gang plow, which usually required four or six horses, could finish three acres per day. Thus, it took several plows about two months to work a 200-acre farm. The only consoling part of the tedious job was the fact that the person seated on the plow could read while the horses kept the plow in position because one horse always walked in the furrow.

"Deaths from farm accidents were relatively small each year but injuries were many. Hardly a season went by without an injury that could disable a farmer for days. Tractors and other more modern farm machines have increased the injury rate even more than when I was a boy. Fortunate for me, I did not sustain any significant injuries on the farm, but I did suffer heat prostration that incapacitated me for a few days. Two of my older brothers and I were loading alfalfa into the hayloft when the incident occurred. The barn was small and did not have a ceiling rack or loading fork. It was a particularly hot day and my brothers decided that they should pitch the hay through the loft door while I dragged the hay into the loft with a pitch fork. We did not realize that without sufficient air circulation, the temperature in the loft soared higher than what it was in the blazing sun outside.

"I felt the heat in no time; the sweat poured off my body in streams. I had carried about two-thirds of the load back from the door of the loft when I felt very weak and dizzy. Then I developed a severe headache and had difficulty with my vision. I was able to make my way to the door of the loft where my brother noticed my condition. Then I collapsed and was helped down. This incident was one of several that spurred my interest in medical school. While I was aware of becoming exceedingly hot, I was more curious to know what was going on inside my body."

George Cole's two-story frame house was typical of the houses built in farming areas all over the United States between the Civil War and the coming of the automobile after the turn of the century, homes immortalized in the paintings of Grant Wood and Grandma Moses. Carpenters generally differentiated the farm house from the barn by putting scroll work under the eaves and by building a front porch with carved wooden posts. Even more than today, the kitchen served as the center of family activity, while the parlor, replete with horsehair-covered furniture, was reserved for special guests, weddings and funerals. The homes were heated by cast-iron stoves, lighted by kerosene lamps and screened in by iron mesh. Before 1900, less than 10 percent of these homes had indoor plumbing. Weekly baths were taken in a wooden washtub and basic bodily functions were cared for in an outhouse. Meals were cooked on a wood or coal stove, and water was hauled or pumped from a nearby well.

Only once was the security of Warren Cole's boyhood home threatened by the waters of the Republican River,

which overflowed its natural boundaries periodically. He remembers the time this way:

"Approximately 180 acres of my father's farm was bottom land and vulnerable to the overflow from the Republican
River, which is considered one of the most destructive of riv-
ers, with roots deep in Colorado. Every three or four years,
the river would rise and inundate vast crop acreage. The
worst flood ever encountered before or since occurred about
1910, when the entire area around our farm was covered by a
raging torrent. As the water line rose, we feared for the
house, which sat on a hill but was endangered nonetheless
because of the unpredictable flow of the mad waters and the
undermining of the banks. Disaster loomed, too, over the
farm land.

"Father became very moody and slept little. This affected me as well as my brothers; we were all aware of the
danger around us. We talked very little about it, however, as
father apparently preferred not to discuss the situation. The
atmosphere about the house was one of deep gloom based on
our fears of tremendous losses. This experience of near disaster brought the family members closer together, a bond
that made us appreciate each other. The Lord must have been
watching over us, for suddenly the waters began to recede,
the river was back to its bank and the actual amount of land
washed out was minimal."

When the river was not raging and threatening the farm,
it was the source of one of the great pleasures of Warren
Cole's entire life—fishing. Anyone who knew him as a adult
was aware of his passion for the art of angling. So devoted
was he to the sport that he even convinced his bride to spend
their honeymoon catching fish.

"When the Republican River was not flooding," he
wrote about his boyhood experiences with a hook and line,
"the water was fairly clear and invited good fishing, the
channel cat being our favorite catch. During the summertime,
we managed to squeeze in a few hours a week, usually on
Sundays, to go fishing. Grasshoppers were used as bait, so
we first had to catch these lively creatures before we could
start. Unless we encountered muddy water, we usually
caught several channel cats and occasionally a carp. Carps

are full of bones, but we ate them for their good taste. A youngster learns early not to swallow the bones and to eat any kind of fish he is able to catch.

"The river was about three-quarters of a mile from the house, a distance that we easily walked to and from. Another body of water, the Stillwater River, spanning about 60 or 70 acres and arching in a semicircular shape, was an offshoot of the Republican and was created when the larger river cut through new soil during a flood. We often went fishing there, although we could only get small mud cats.

"I recall a most frightening incident that happened on the Republican River when I was about 10 years old. My brother and I had surrounded some stumps with a seine in the hope of catching some big fish in water that was about four feet deep. Suddenly I felt something hit me in the abdomen with such force that it almost knocked me over. I quickly clambered out of the water and onto the bank and warned my brother to do the same, so sure was I that an alligator was in there. Of course, my brother did not panic, knowing that alligators have never been found so far north. I finally got back into the water and, working together, we cornered the huge fish against the net and flipped it into a gunnysack. It turned out to be a 48-pound channel cat and a welcome addition to our diet."

Such idyllic scenes of childhood innocence are indicative of a life that has virtually vanished from the American landscape along with the family farms that were the soul of it. Warren was fortunate to grow up on a farm when he did, for the period from 1897 to 1920 has been called the Golden Age of American Agriculture, a period when farm income was relatively high. After that, a post-war depression hit farmers in the 1920s, and the Great Depression devastated rural areas as well as cities in the 1930s.

His father had to be a shrewd farmer to keep the farm growing and prospering in the period before the turn of the century, which was marked by depressions, high freight rates, tight credit, low farm prices and the rising cost of goods and services. But in the first two decades of the 20th century, both the U.S. population and world trade increased, farm prices rose faster than industrial prices and prosperity came to the family farm.

The boy that emerged during the years on that Kansas farm was lean and wiry, not unlike his father, and quiet and shy. He showed a capacity for long and hard work, a characteristic he was to maintain throughout his life, and an aptitude for keen observation, a trait that led him to be a brilliant medical researcher. Farm life kept him innocent and unsophisticated, yet imbued him with the wholesome American values of the importance of work, family and education. During those years, what Dr. Cole refers to as his character was forged by a plowshare and tempered by the heat of the family fire.

THE ONE-ROOM SCHOOLHOUSE

W hen the farmers settled the western plains, they built their houses, established their churches and set up school districts that provided free elementary and high school education for all. The farm home, however, was considered the center of education as well as family life, and children were taught how to make handicrafts and given lessons in catechism and moral living at their own hearths.

The role of the one-room schoolhouse, which dominated elementary education in rural areas well into the 20th century, was to provide the basics of the three Rs, not complete preparation for life. In 1912, author Warren Wilson, in his book *Evolution of the Country Community*, wrote: "The farmer of the day relied for his son and daughter not upon trained skill, but upon native abilities, sterling character, independence, and industry. Of all these, the household not the school is the source. So that the one-room country school was satisfactory to those who created it."

Typically the schoolhouse was a small structure made of clapboard and built on a corner lot close to the main highway. The children, often more than 100 crowded into one room, sat on benches facing the master's high desk and a wood stove. The schools taught the rudiments of reading, writing and arithmetic, along with a smattering of geography and history. Learning by rote was the common method of teaching. Sometimes all of the children read aloud at once or recited from memory in concert. Spelling was taught by a technique called spelling down, in which the children stood in a long line and were sent to the end of the line if they incorrectly spelled a word given by the teacher.

Shortly after his mother died in 1904, Warren Cole started school when he was still five years old. "It was a mile-and-a-quarter walk to the school," he wrote in his retirement years, "which was one large room with a pot-bellied stove around which, in winter, the students sat on benches. I recall that the major discomfort was in getting to school—the lengthy walks in the mornings in the bitter cold. Despite overshoes, ear muffs, mittens and long underwear, there never seemed to be sufficient clothing to withstand the elements. Instinctively, we developed a genuine concern for one another, checking for any signs of frostbite or undue danger.

"The school, with an enrollment of 25 to 35 students, had only one teacher. During our study periods, we learned not to be interrupted by the constant sounds and recitations from the other student groups. As is often the case, one remembers incidents occurring during childhood more vividly than events of more recent date. I can recall practically all the teachers of those early days, perhaps because they were good instructors. The one I remember very well is Mr. Terwilliger, who administered my first spanking at about age six. He was very strict about enforcing the 'no whispering' rule. One day, a student sitting in back of me asked me a lengthy question that necessitated more than a yes or no reply. Mr. Terwilliger turned around just in time to catch me answering my friend; he immediately called me to his side to be reprimanded.

"The spanking did not hurt physically, but it wounded my feelings, which was the intent. Nevertheless, it makes me shudder to think what would happen to today's teacher who would dare to whip a child! Teachers in my day used a switch or a rule; I consider such deserved punishment effective in instilling discipline, especially as it applied to me. I received the spanking through the fault of my friend; however, I felt that I should not attempt to explain, 'My friend asked the question which led to the whisper.' Now and then it is preferable to assume the blame for another.

"I would presume that today educators would condemn the one-room school house as an antiquated and ineffective method of teaching. I received my entire pre-high school training in one room, and I see many advantages to it. In the first place, I congratulate those teachers for delivering effective education for the majority of students. Probably the mentally retarded children did not get all they deserved because the teachers simply did not have the time to give them extra help.

"The teacher showed a lot of ingenuity in arranging and hearing classes throughout the day. He or she had to spend the entire day hearing classes, and this gave the teacher ample opportunity to find out which students were superior and which inferior to the others. The superior student was given the opportunity to move ahead from grade to grade faster than the modern method. For example, I was pushed ahead and finished grade school in six years. I entered high school at the age of twelve. Of course, I had to take an examination given by the county to determine if I was ready for high school.

"I never felt that the student was given a really good opportunity to spend whatever extra time he had on something worthwhile. Our teacher encouraged the students to go to the library, which consisted of two shelves of books in a small bookcase. I had read most of these books, and I am not convinced they were well chosen for the student to spend his extra time on. My father had a similar library of about two shelves, and I had read most of these too. I can remember that when we were out of something to do, we would raise our hand and ask for the privilege of going to the library. The teacher would always ask, 'Have you completed your lessons for tomorrow's classes?' Unless we had, we could not go to the library."

Spelling contests among children in neighboring school districts were a popular diversion for adults in the winter months. Dr. Cole remembered a county-wide contest that he participated in and that taught him a lesson for life. "The idea of having spelling contests in school was popular, and

most schools had a spelling bee of one type or another sometime during the year. I recall one year that the county school
system proposed a spelling contest throughout the county. I
was chosen along with one other student to represent our
school (the Sherwood School). Two student representatives
each were chosen from 15 or 20 other schools, and we all
went to a nearby town, Morganville, for the contest. There
were perhaps 30 or 35 students representing several town-
ships. The superintendent of the Morganville schools was the
host, but a teacher from another township was chosen as
moderator. He selected the words to be spelled by the various contestants from a large spelling book.

"After an hour or two of the contest, only two students
were left—a student from Morganville was one and I was the
other. I recall that the words chosen by the moderator from
the outside township were fairly chosen. However, at one
point, the moderator had to excuse himself, perhaps to go to
the little boys' room, and he turned the choice of words over
to the superintendent of Morganville schools. Almost immediately, I realized that I was being given the more difficult
words.

"The other student then tripped up on a fairly simple
word—balloon. He left out one 'l'. I recognized his error immediately and thought to myself, 'This gives me the township championship.' But not so. The Morganville superintendent had other ideas. Immediately he said to the boy,
'No, you misunderstood the word. The word is balloon.' The
student got the tip immediately and respelled the word cor-
rectly.

"A half a dozen things flashed through my mind. My
student friend missed the word but was given another
chance—that is unfair. What can I do? Anything? I could politely say, 'He missed the word. The contest is over.' But the
Morganville teacher continued. He gave me the next word,
and it was a hard one. I quickly decided that it would be entirely improper for me to criticize the Morganville superintendent. So I could do nothing about the situation, which I
could now see was hopeless for me. Naturally I became a bit
depressed, and careless, knowing that I had no chance. The
obvious thing happened. I missed a word and the contest

was over.

"I learned a lot from this incident. Now and then throughout my life things were going to happen which were beyond my control. I must recognize this and not beat my brains in with a useless effort to correct the situation. I could see that, in these circumstances, it was important to realize that the situation was hopeless and learn to control my emotions.

"It so happened that this incident did not affect my chances of winning the county championship because two from each township were chosen to go to the county contest. My young Morganville friend and I were appointed to go to the finals at the county high school. We went, but we were both spelled down by more efficient spellers."

At an early age, young Warren exhibited a love of learning and a curiosity about the physical world about him that prepared him for the study of medicine. However, he points to one incident in his boyhood that became the deciding factor in choosing to become a doctor. When he was about eight years old, he came down with an intermittent fever that persisted for several weeks. His father called a local doctor who had a large country practice. About three times a week, this doctor made his rounds of the countryside. He would drive 15 or 20 miles seeing patients along the way, then a driver would meet him with a new team of horses and he would continue for another 15 miles to the end of the day.

After the doctor examined Warren, he and George Cole went off to an adjacent room where Warren could overhear their conversation. "Doctor, what's the matter with my boy?" George Cole asked with grave concern. The memory of Sophia's death still haunted him.

"He has typhoid malaria," replied the doctor with an air of certainty, although he might have known there was no such disease and was indicating that the fever resembled a cross between the two ailments.

Warren Cole was shocked to hear the diagnosis. Years later he recounted his reaction: "At that time I was a voracious reader. I had read all the books in my father's library, which was contained on one shelf in a small bookcase and consisted of perhaps 20 to 25 books. One of the books was en-

titled *Dr. Pierce's Golden Medical Discoveries*. It described all
the diseases known at that time. (Undulant fever, which is
probably what I had, was unknown at the time.) I had read
about typhoid fever and malaria, but there was no disease
called typhoid malaria. I said to myself, 'That doctor is the
best in town and making good money. If he is so poorly informed yet so successful, there is room for me. I'm going to
be a doctor.'"

Warren Cole was one of the fortunate ones of the time
who was smart enough and motivated enough to move on to
high school, in September of 1910. Many farm children of his
era thought only of working the land and were content to get
the basics of education in elementary school or, worse yet,
not even stay in school long enough to get an eighth-grade
diploma. In fact, a survey of rural schools taken between 1906
and 1913 in Colorado showed that a mere 22 percent of the
64,385 children enrolled in those schools graduated from
eighth grade.

High school, as we know it today, was pretty much an
invention of the 20th century. As late as 1890, a paltry seven
percent of the nation's children aged 14 to 17 were enrolled in
all of the public high schools and private secondary schools
across the United States. The free public high school was a
distinctly American invention. In the last half of the 19th century, America had developed, through a combination of private philanthropy and public land grants, a comprehensive
system of colleges and universities. Educators began to recognize the need for preparatory institutions beyond the elementary level that would be open to all citizens and would
ready students for a college education. The change came in
1899 when John Dewey, the apostle of modern education,
published his book *School and Society* and urged that schools
take over the role of the disappearing family farm by pre-
paring children for the new tasks of life in a changing world.

Dr. Cole remembered that he was the first one up in the
morning when he was going to high school and that he usually fixed breakfast for the whole family. In order to get to
Clay County High School by horse and buggy by 9:00 am
when school started, he had to leave home at 7:30. Before he
left, he placed the family's breakfast on the back of the stove

and fired the stove in the living room in the winter. "When my brother and I were in high school together," he wrote in later years, "he would attend to the barn chores while I did the cooking. Later, I had to do both. This routine, month after month, no doubt helped to shape my own character.

"My three older brothers attended high school before I got there. They drove the six miles to Clay Center in a horse-pulled buggy. My eldest brother, Perry, who was eight years my senior, graduated from high school and later obtained a degree in civil engineering from the University of Kansas. He had no difficulty finding work and spent his life doing various types of engineering jobs. In his later years he built roads in Nebraska.

"When it came my time to attend high school, my brother Irvin had transferred to the State Agricultural College in Manhattan to devote his time to farm studies. Cecil was starting his third year of high school at the time, so we drove the route together, a six mile drive.

"The winters in Kansas were severe; the intense cold provoked high winds from the flat plains. The temperature often dropped below zero and accumulated snowdrifts sometimes rose five or six feet deep in some sections. About a quarter of a mile from our house, the road that led to school ran between two hedges. Snowdrifts there often made the road impassable for man, beast, buggy or wagon. To get through this area, we would have to take down a fence and go through a neighbor's wheat field to reach a passable road. En route to the school, we tried to keep the buggy behind hedges and away from the wind, which could easily freeze exposed skin.

"When I was in my third year of high school, I had to go alone. During this period, I was driving a horse that was blind. We still used her because of her remarkable stamina and her ability to trot, although at a slow pace, between home and school. This extraordinary horse was unusually intelligent; she knew every bump in the road over the six miles we traveled. You might say she learned it the hard way. We would steer her away from the bumps, but she was usually able to avoid them without any guidance. And she automatically stopped at the crossroads as if to say, 'I'm not going across until you assure me there is no cross traffic.'

"The horse was kept in a rented barn not far from school. Cecil and I would go there at noon to feed her and eat our lunch. She was like a camel, not requiring any water after her morning drink at the watering tank until she returned home in the late afternoon. I remember a few times when she got stuck in the snowdrifts and I had to get out and extricate both horse and buggy. This did not happen very often, however, because we would check the first quarter mile when the snow was drifting, and if it appeared to be too high, down would come the neighbor's fence and into his field we drove. Kansas farmers were friendly and cooperative, but we always made sure that the fence was replaced, so thankful were we to be accorded the favor.

"Youngsters are strange individuals who apparently have similar characteristics everywhere. For some strange reason, we seldom put on our overshoes for the buggy ride, even though the cold was so intense that our toes were often almost frozen. We covered ourselves with a bearskin rug, but it was really not warm enough. Once in a while, we placed a large comforter over the bearskin for added warmth. Why we did not use both covers on all cold days, I do not understand.

"I dwell on the subject of driving to school because it represented one of the many hardships of the country. For the three or four months of winter each year, the cold was so extreme that we were quite miserable on those trips. Yet I am sure that this ordeal helped us children from taking things for granted. It was a condition we had to endure, and we tolerated it without complaint. That day is now long past. Today a roomy bus drives up to pick up the students and transport them to school."

At the time that Warren Cole was in high school, 1910–1914, The University of Kansas set the standards for accredited county high schools. The curriculum included English, mathematics, foreign languages, physical sciences, biological sciences and history. Warren remembered being strong in sciences and math but weak in languages, especially Latin. Socially, "I was quiet and a bit slow in mingling with other students," he said. "I realized I was bashful but couldn't help it—to my detriment, I think. It lasted up through college days to some extent."

Long before Warren Cole had finished high school, he wanted to study medicine. His curiosity about the physical nature of things and his experience with ineffective doctors—both during his mother's operation on the kitchen table and his own bout with fever—led to a conviction that he could become a better doctor than the ones he knew, and that the world needed better doctors. Ironically, it was his mother's death that led to the biggest obstacle to his becoming a physician, especially a surgeon.

Warren's father had grown to dislike and mistrust the medical profession, and he strongly objected to Warren's goal. His opposition was an exception to his usual attitude toward his sons. "Father seldom argued with us boys," Dr. Cole later recounted, "and never were we whipped. His loud voice was his most effective weapon by which he maintained stern discipline in the family."

Although George Cole voiced his objections strenuously, Warren persisted "without unpleasant words." Ultimately, his father gave his reluctant approval but he was never enthusiastic about the idea. "My father had great strength and love for his children," he recalled. "We didn't know it then, but looking back now, I can see it. He wasn't demonstrative in exhibiting his feelings, but he treated us all with true respect. He was also a bashful individual, like me. He hated the doctors and didn't want me to mingle with them. In spite of that feeling, however, he finally gave up his antagonism and told me to go ahead, which pleased me very much."

What Warren Cole knew of doctors and medicine was limited to what he saw in his home town of Clay Center. There were seven or eight doctors in town when he was in high school; all were general practitioners and some performed some minor surgery. A boarding house had by then been put to use as Clay Center's only hospital. "The doctors of that time didn't really know very much about their field," Dr. Cole commented in later years. "The things that some of them did would just make you shiver to death. They might make a diagnosis of a fracture and treat the patient for fracture whereas it might not have been that. Rest was the main therapy for patients in the hospital, although the doctors administered a lot of pills. I don't know what they all were, but cathartics were common. A lot of people died in the hospital and everybody feared it. There were no antibiotics then and a bad infection would kill you."

Since money was tight, the University of Kansas was the logical choice for college. At 16, Warren Cole was the youngest person ever to enter the university to that date (he was actually 15 when he was accepted). The school offered a BS degree in medicine, which required that he undertake two years of premedical college studies and two years of lectures and lab work in the medical school. In September of 1914, Warren Cole, small, young and shy, headed for Lawrence, Kansas, and a career that would take him into medical history books.

SECTION TWO:

❧

MEDICAL TRAINING

CHAPTER 4

❧

THE MAKING OF A DOCTOR

W ith the rise of scientific medicine just before the turn of the century came a move toward reform of the nation's medical schools. Throughout the late 19th century, medical educators began to reject the formalism that had dominated the teaching of medicine and attempted to abandon dry lectures and sterile textbook learning for laboratory experience and bedside discovery. John Dewey led the rebellion against traditional methods of general education, and medical educators quickly followed. The teachers of medicine of that period were faced with the shock of an information explosion as real as any we face today. "The time has gone by when one mind can encompass all which has been ascertained in the medical sciences," maintained William Welch, a pioneer in medical education at Johns Hopkins, in 1886.

The quintessential modern medical school, and the model for all that followed, was the Johns Hopkins Medical School, which opened its doors in the fall of 1893 after Baltimore philanthropist Johns Hopkins left $7 million in his will for the establishment of a university, a hospital and a medical school to unite them. Under a system devised by the first professor of medicine at Hopkins, William Osler, who has been called the greatest American clinical teacher, every

third and fourth year medical student used the wards of the
Johns Hopkins Hospital as a classroom and participated in
the care of real patients.

The distinguished Hopkins faculty—John Abel, William
Halsted, William Howell, Howard Kelly, Franklin Mall, William Osler and William Welch—led the way to a new era in
medical education that saw the introduction of entrance requirements, a nine-month school term, the four-year medical
course, compulsory oral and written examinations, and an
expanded curriculum that included instruction in anatomy,
physiology, physiological chemistry, pathology, pharmacology and bacteriology. In addition, the Hopkins pioneers
increased the scope of clinical teaching beyond the traditional
courses in medicine, surgery and obstetrics to new courses in
gynecology, pediatrics, dermatology, genitourinary diseases,
laryngology, ophthalmology, otology, psychiatry and hygiene. Through all of these changes, the role of the student
was transformed from passive listener to active learner in the
laboratory and clerkship.

But despite the efforts of these giants of education, medical schools across the country were slow to change and uneven in their development of progressive educational methods. By 1910, the standards of medical teaching had emerged,
but among the nation's 148 undergraduate and postgraduate
schools of medicine—almost half of the total number of medical schools in the entire world—were some of the greatest
and some of the worst schools anywhere. In the first decade
of the 20th century, however, medical reform found its greatest champion in Abraham Flexner, a professional educator,
who in June 1910 issued his now-famous report, *Medical Education in the United States and Canada*, as Bulletin Number
Four of the Carnegie Foundation for the Advancement of
Teaching.

Carrying the full endorsement of both the Carnegie
Foundation and the American Medical Association, the Flexner report was a classic in muckraking journalism whose
ringing phrases and carefully detailed charges galvanized
public concern for the quality of medical education. Outspoken and aggressive, Flexner, a graduate of Johns Hopkins
who pursued graduate study at Harvard, began his project in

December of 1908 by traveling to each of the 155 medical schools in the United States and Canada and writing about what he saw. He evaluated the schools on the basis of their entrance requirements, the size and training of their faculty, their financial resources, their laboratory facilities and their clinical facilities. Throughout his report, he expressed scorn for didactic instruction and held up the university-affiliated medical school based on the Johns Hopkins system, rather than the proprietary schools, as the ideal model.

Flexner's report dealt a lethal blow to a group of proprietary medical schools in Kansas, including the University Medical College, the oldest of the proprietary schools. He described virtually all of the schools in the Greater Kansas City area as "utterly wretched," and he wrote that the dissecting room at Kansas Medical College in Topeka was "indescribably filthy; it contained, in addition to necessary tables, a single, badly hacked cadaver, and was simultaneously used as a chicken yard."

Flexner saw the University of Kansas School of Medicine as the only hope for the future of medical education in the state but found the school poorly organized, underfunded by the state and sadly divided into two campuses. "This institution has shown the desire to provide instruction of high grade by raising its entrance requirements until they now call for two years of college work," he wrote, "but it did not realize that it was incumbent upon it to improve facilities and instruction at the same time."

The state legislative act of 1864 that established the University of Kansas foresaw a medical school as part of the university, but it was not until 1905 that a full four-year program evolved. In 1879, a one-year preparatory course in medicine was set up at the university's campus in Lawrence, but groups of physicians in various larger cities wanted to woo the medical school to their area. In 1894, Dr. Simon Bell of Rosedale, a suburb of Kansas City, offered the university land and money totaling $75,000 in value on the provision that a hospital be built in Rosedale and that the medical school provide at least clinical teaching there. Meanwhile, in 1899, a second year was added to the preparatory medical courses offered at Lawrence.

The board of regents and the state legislature failed to act on Simon Bell's offer until Bell promised them another $25,000 in land and cash in 1904. Suddenly and quickly, the university acquired the students, faculty and facilities of three existing medical schools in Kansas City—the College of Physicians and Surgeons of Kansas City, Kansas; the Medico-Chirurgical College; and the Kansas City Medical College of Missouri—and inaugurated a four-year medical school. The first two years of study, consisting of science and laboratory courses, remained at Lawrence, while the last two years of clinical instruction were conducted at Rosedale after the Eleanor Taylor Bell Memorial Hospital was completed in 1906.

The state legislature gave only lukewarm support to the Rosedale facility and many of the state's physicians resented the fact that the majority of the faculty at Rosedale were Missouri doctors. The hospital was small, the facilities inadequate, the budget scanty, and the university was able to exert little authority over unsalaried faculty with outside practices who gave merely a small token of their time to the medical school.

By the time Warren Cole entered college at the University of Kansas in Lawrence in 1914, the Flexner report had had some effect on turning things around at the medical school. A new dean was chosen in 1911—Dr. Samuel Crumbine, who had made a name for himself waging campaigns for pure food laws as secretary of the state board of health—but the money needed to improve the facility at Rosedale was not available. Eventually the university did get the funds necessary to turn the school of medicine into a first-rate institution, but in the early years the medical school suffered greatly from careless planning and poor funding.

While the clinical instruction at Rosedale flailed along, the quality of the scientific departments at Lawrence was enhanced by a faculty that boasted some excellent professors who acquired national and even worldwide reputations: Lucien Sayre in pharmacology, E.H.S. Bailey in chemistry, Marshall Barber and Noble P. Sherwood in bacteriology, and George Ellet Coghill in anatomy. In 1912, however, a half-year of medical studies was transferred to the Rosedale campus, leaving only the first one and one-half years of the medical school at Lawrence.

"I can well remember," Dr. Cole said years later, "that my first year in school cost a total of $320. I lived in a small room in a boarding house that cost $6 a month. I had an aunt in Lawrence who helped me find it. My dad couldn't afford any more. And I joined what was called an eating club in the boarding house. The cost of the meals was divided up at the end of each week and each person paid his share. I paid, on average, about $3.75 a week for food."

A photograph of Warren Cole taken in November of 1914 shows him sitting at his desk in the tiny room of the boarding house on Mississippi Avenue in Lawrence, with an eyeshade on his head and a bare electric bulb hanging above him. There is a small bookcase in one corner and two college pennants hanging on the wall behind him—one for Kansas, the other for Nebraska—along with two tennis rackets. A ukulele stands propped against the wall.

In 1916, the year Warren began his studies in the medical school at Lawrence, a committee appointed by the state legislature recommended the abolition of the Rosedale plant, arguing that the Rosedale school was isolated from the university, that it faced stiff competition from the schools in St. Louis and Chicago, and that it was enormously expensive to maintain for the poor results it achieved. "The university had practically nothing in the way of a medical school when I was there," Dr. Cole recalled. "They had one small building where we had our anatomy, physiology and other medical classes. Even the students knew that medical training in Kansas was not very effective."

Warren helped pay for his medical school expenses by working during the summer months. Since the dean of the medical school was also head of the state board of health, there was extensive cooperation between the two entities in research and educational projects. Warren Cole spent one summer working for the public health service on one such project. He described the experience in this way:

"When I was attending early medical school in Lawrence, the Kansas State Public Health Service offered me a very attractive job for the summer. I cannot remember whether I was a freshman or a sophomore in medicine, but I believe bacteriology was not taught at Kansas until the first half of the sophomore year. Since this job involved testing water for typhoid contamination, it must have been in the sophomore year or else I would not have been able to do the water-testing. I recall very distinctly that we had an experiment in our bacteriology laboratory class which involved culturing water for *E. coli* bacteria growth as evidence of typhoid contamination.

"I cannot remember how the public health officer got in touch with me because the second half of the second year of study was held in Rosedale, and I believe that we went directly home from Rosedale, not returning to Lawrence. At any rate, the public health officer contacted Dr. Sherwood, our bacteriology professor (who was a fine teacher and a splendid gentleman), for a bright, mature and conscientious student to do the work. I am grateful to my bacteriology teacher for a fine compliment. Bright—I don't know because I missed A.O.A. [Alpha Omega Alpha, an honor society for medical students] by a fraction. Mature—I'm not sure about that because I was only 19 years of age, and the youngest man in the class by far. And I was a country boy at that. I had not learned many of the tricks of life and the world yet. But that may be what my bacteriology professor was looking for—minimal contamination.

"At the request of the public health officer, I reported to Eldorado, Kansas, an oil town of about 15,000 population at the time. They had had a severe typhoid epidemic there the year before, and the officials had enough evidence to suspect the water wells as the source. Thousands of people had their own water wells because they only had to drive down about 30 feet to reach water, and there were no rocks to go through. The city water service was relatively new and expensive to use.

"I was told that I would find a laboratory and supplies to culture the water at a certain address on the second story of a warehouse. There I found a steam sterilizer, Petri dishes, a huge supply of agar and other things needed for my culturing work. I began assembling the material and sterilizing the water bottles. I also found a map of water wells in the area.

"After culturing water from the various wells, I was supposed to put a tag on the side of each well to indicate how they tested. I had been working only a few days when I learned from two public health nurses I had become friends with that the people who owned the wells did not like me because they suspected I was going to put kerosene into their wells if the wells tested positive for *E. coli*. I assured the owners I spoke to that I was not going to do that. But I did not realize how widespread the talk about me and my kerosene was; otherwise I would have placed a note in the town paper.

"For many weeks, I continued uneventfully with my testing. Then one day I narrowly escaped being bitten by a vicious dog. I had just placed a 'positive' tag on a man's well when a huge bulldog came at me from the shadows of the house with its mouth open and growling. I recognized his intent and quickly picked up my hammer and box of bottles and retreated to the street. The owner of the house came out and began cursing me. Just then, I let the heavy box of water bottles drop just in front of the charging dog. At the same time, I warned the owner to call the dog off, but he didn't. Then a strange thing happened. The dog stopped in his tracks. His mouth closed, he stopped growling and he waited there, watching me closely. Something gave that dog a message that he was in possible danger from the water. I don't know what it was, but as I reached the sidewalk next door, the dog retreated. I don't know how he got the message, but I was very grateful and went on my way.

"Only a few days after that incident I received a letter from my boss saying we would have to stop the project. He did not say why. Was it because the city manager was receiving so many complaints or because the health office ran out of money? I don't know. At any rate, I had been employed nicely for two and a half months.

"I had a month left before I had to go back to medical school, and it happened that the local health officer lost his helper on another project. He was delighted when I became available and I spent the rest of the summer working with him. I mention this because something happened on the second project that made a big impression on me. At that time, milk bottles were just coming into use and the local health officer was trying to get restaurants to buy milk in small bottles and dispense milk from the bottles. The hotel in Eldorado had a small lunch counter in it where I frequently ate breakfast. At that time, I often drank a glass of milk with breakfast.

"I was certain I had seen the hotel manager dip my glass into a large can of milk to fill it, a practice that was not completely hygienic. I told the health officer about the way the manager served milk because he had asked me to look for such errors; a pure milk law had just been passed locally and he wanted to test it. My boss said, 'Good, let's go over there in the morning and serve a ticket on him.' So we served him with the proper ticket and took him to court in a day or two. It was a very small matter, I confess, but you must start small. If we could correct the hotel's practice, we could start to get the effect of the law that we wanted.

"Everybody showed up in court on the assigned date, and after a certain amount of routine questioning, the judge turned to me and said, 'Mr. Cole, are you absolutely sure you saw Mr. Jones actually dip the milk out of a large can into a glass?' The importance that the judge attached to the question startled me. As I thought back to the incident two or three days previously, it dawned on me that as the hotel manager had opened the large ice box to get the milk, I had turned to the lunchroom door to greet an acquaintance who came in. When I turned my head back, the glass of milk was sitting in front of me. No, I had not actually seen the transfer of milk, but it was obvious it had occurred as I suspected. When I hesitated in my response and indicated that I was not absolutely sure I had seen the motion of the manager, the judge said gently, 'Not sure? Case dismissed.'

"I apologized to my boss, who said, 'Don't worry, we have made our point. I predict the manager will now abide by the law.' And when I returned to the lunchroom, I discovered that the manager was now serving milk from small bottles. But I too had certainly learned a lesson from this incident. One must always be accurate and one must always make an effort to keep inaccuracy to a minimum."

Disappointed with what the University of Kansas had to offer at the Rosedale school, young Warren and some of his friends were impressed by advertising literature they received showing much better clinical facilities at the Washington University School of Medicine in St. Louis. He and about seven of his medical school chums were swayed by what they saw and heard about the St. Louis institution and decided to finish medical school there.

While Warren was still at Rosedale, the great influenza pandemic of 1918-1919 broke out. The first wave of the outbreak started in the United States in early spring of 1918; it was regarded as mild and mortality from it was not unusually high. As many as 40 percent of the victims were under 35 years old, and as is true of most flu epidemics, the majority of deaths were in old people. The second wave came in the fall of 1918, starting in Europe, and it was the most spectacular outbreak of any disease to have occurred for hundreds of years. The United States had entered World War I in 1917, and the movement of our troops into Europe in 1918 is cited as a way that the disease was spread from America. An unusual feature of the second wave was that about half the deaths were among people in the 20 to 40 age group. The final wave in early 1919 was less severe, but the total effect of the three outbreaks was devastating. The estimated death toll was 15 to 25 million people worldwide—one of the greatest plagues ever to strike the human race. Most of the deaths were due to streptococcal pneumonia occasioned by influenza.

Dr. Cole remembered being sick in the first wave of infection. "I had that flu but a mild case of it in the spring. Later that year, at Washington University, George Dock, who was our professor of medicine and a very brilliant man, kept the sick students segregated so the healthy ones wouldn't be exposed, but the epidemic didn't shut down our class work at all."

Working in another part of the country in the spring of 1918, at Camp Lee in Petersburg, Virginia, was a 36-year-old Army captain who had recently been appointed to the Empyema Commission, a committee of health professionals brought together by the Surgeon General of the Army and charged with the task of studying and devising ways to treat empyema, a buildup of pus in the cavity surrounding the lungs and one complication of pneumonia brought on by influenza. The captain was Dr. Evarts A. Graham, who was later to become professor of surgery at Washington University School of Medicine and the greatest influence on Warren Cole's academic life. His astute research on the treatment of empyema won him professional honors and the chairmanship of the department of surgery—and helped save many lives in the second wave of the flu epidemic of 1918.

Because Warren Cole was young and small as a student at the University of Kansas, he did not go out for college sports, and because he was shy, he was not distracted by a busy social life. And so he studied, long and hard, and made the most of what Kansas had to offer academically. His choice of Washington University School of Medicine was a wise one not only because it provided him with superior medical training but also because it led him to one of the most fortuitous matchings of resident and chief in the annals of modern surgery—Warren Cole and Evarts Graham.

Chapter 5

ॐ

The Modern Man of Medicine

As a medical student, Warren Cole was exempt from service in the Armed Forces during World War I. However, medical students were required to be in the reserves and to train for military combat. Thus, Cole and his classmates were outfitted with uniforms and rifles and made to practice military maneuvers every morning between seven and eight o'clock on the campus of Washington University School of Medicine.

When the armistice was signed on November 11, 1918, there were celebrations throughout the western world. "Peace was signed and all hell broke loose in celebrations in all the towns across the United States," Dr. Cole remembered. The mayor of St. Louis wanted to stage a military parade in honor of the occasion, but the servicemen had not returned home from fighting yet and so he could not find anyone in uniform for the parade. "The mayor finally discovered that out at the medical school was a company of 150 men, and he asked our lieutenant, 'Is your company fully equipped?'

'Yes,' the lieutenant replied, 'we even have bayonets.'

'Put them on!' the mayor ordered, 'and come downtown for a parade. We want a parade.'

"I'll never forget that day because it was five miles from the medical school to downtown St. Louis, and while we had practiced our maneuvers every day, we were somewhat green physically. And so our lieutenant said, 'Boys, it's five miles down there, but I'll give you a rest halfway there.' We marched all the way, resting after about two and one-half miles, with our guns and bayonets fixed.

"As we were walking, a couple of little boys began to follow alongside me, and one of them said to the other, 'Gee, I bet they were in the war just yesterday. They just came over from France.' I had to hold back a laugh. I didn't have the heart to tell him that we hadn't been to war at all but that we were grinding away in medical school."

Even before he had arrived in St. Louis, Warren Cole was contacted by the medical fraternity at Washington University to join the group and live in its campus housing. "The fraternity was so anxious to get students into their building that they contacted me and some of the others when they found out we were coming," he recalled. "I can't remember whether I moved into the fraternity's dormitory first or the Nu Sigma Nu house, but I lived in both places. They were both about two or three blocks away from the medical center."

One of his first friends at his new medical school was Alton Ochsner, who in 1927 became professor of surgery and chairman of the department at Tulane University School of Medicine and in 1942 helped found and served as director of surgery of the Ochsner Clinic and Ochsner Foundation Hospital in New Orleans. At Dr. Cole's retirement party from the University of Illinois in 1966, Dr. Ochsner fondly remembered their meeting: "I remember very well a day in September 1918 when two country boys arrived in St. Louis. Warren had had his first two years in medicine at the University of Kansas and I had had my first two years at the University of South Dakota. And I can assure you that no two boys knew less about city life than Warren and I did. With that beginning, a friendship has developed which is probably as close as any two people can have."

During their lifetimes, the two country boys set the world of surgery and medical education on fire. Alton Ochsner was a pioneer in promoting the ideals of group practice and prepaid health care from salaried doctors, which are thoroughly modern concepts that have revolutionized medicine in the last half of the 20th century. But perhaps his greatest contribution was in establishing the link between cigarette smoking and lung cancer.

In an interview in 1981, shortly before his death, Alton Ochsner described a time in 1919 when his professor of medicine at Washington U., Dr. George Dock, had his class witness the autopsy of a patient who had died of lung cancer. The condition was so rare, the professor told the class, that the students would probably never see another case as long as they lived. "I didn't see another case for 17 years, until 1936. Then I saw nine cases in six months. An epidemic. There had to be a cause. The patients were all men who smoked heavily and began smoking in World War I. I researched the history of smoking and found that very few cigarettes were consumed before the first world war."

Dr. Ochsner presented his first research findings on smoking and cancer in 1938, but it took him years to convince a skeptical scientific community. Even when he was president of the American Cancer Society in 1950, the society's chief biostatistician fought him over the causal link. For more than 40 years he waged an indefatigable assault on the use of tobacco in 82 scientific articles, four books, and hundreds of interviews, films and speeches around the world. For many of those years, he was virtually alone in his campaign.

Warren Cole remembered Alton Ochsner as "a great fellow and a great man. We lived in the same fraternity house at Washington University. He was not a shy person at all but he never wanted to prevaricate, always wanted to speak to the truth. He was always a fair individual who never pulled any dirty tricks on anybody. That made him popular. Everybody liked him. He was an attractive young fellow and a brilliant lad. He appreciated friendship, and he and I were very close friends throughout our entire careers. In medical school we would take our girlfriends out to dinner together. We never studied together because I don't feel that you can study effectively with someone else."

Both Alton and Warren had come to St. Louis with two years of preclinical medical education behind them, anxious to begin seeing patients during clinical rounds in hospital wards. Both had benefited from the reforms that swept through American medical schools after Flexner's report and were trained as modern men of medicine. By the time they had entered preclinical training, a curriculum of graded courses in the medical sciences had replaced the didactic lectures scorned by Flexner. Students advanced through the four years of medical school after passing rigid examinations; those who failed individual courses were allowed to take the exams again or to repeat the year, but those who failed examinations in about half of their courses were asked to leave.

The first year of study—devoted to gross and microscopic anatomy, biochemistry and physiology—was a grueling experience for anybody who did not have a facile memory. Students spent almost half their time in anatomy dissecting rooms with a copy of Gray's *Anatomy* in hand, trying to match nerves, muscles, bones and organs with the appropriate Latin name. Biochemistry, a subject fast becoming recognized as the basic foundation of scientific medicine, dealt primarily with nutrition and metabolism. Most first-year students found the study of physiology the most exciting because it most closely approximated treating living patients by allowing them to operate on anesthetized animals and observe human physiological changes in their classmates.

The second-year courses usually included pathology, bacteriology, pharmacology and an introduction to clinical medicine. The last half of the second year included a course in physical diagnosis that taught history-taking and other simple clinical tasks. Warren Cole had gone to Rosedale, Kansas, for this part of his training. The student was given a stethoscope and clean white coat and sent into the open wards to look and listen for signs of disease and gradually overcome any sense of insecurity. This was his or her first taste of patient care.

The last two years of medical school were based on the British system of clinical clerkship, which exposes the student to the care provided by a variety of medical specialists at work in outpatient clinics and hospital wards. Under close supervision by their clinical professors, medical students were allowed to take part in the actual care of real patients. It is a system that is still used today because it has the virtue of never going out of date—the diseases and treatment methods reflect what is prevalent at the time and not some outdated textbook.

At Washington University, Warren and Alton had the facilities of Barnes Hospital and St. Louis Children's Hospital as their clinical training grounds. Their professor of medicine was the great George Dock, whom Warren Cole called "one of the top ten internists of the time." Alton Ochsner subsequently served his medical internship and assistant residency under George Dock at Barnes Hospital in 1920 and 1921.

Dock was of the new breed of clinical scientists who were now being attracted to the medical schools. Unlike the part-time clinical professors who preceded them, they were trained laboratory investigators who had acquired additional scientific training in physiology, biochemistry and immunology as a background to investigating the fundamental mechanisms of disease. And they aspired to careers in teaching and research rather than in private practice. Although most of the clinical professors saw patients, their primary goal was to study disease in the laboratory.

It was George Dock who influenced both Warren and Alton to take an additional year of medical training as interns in internal medicine, no matter what their ultimate career choice would be. Dock often told students of the advantages of taking additional hospital training rather than going straight into practice from medical school. The student would be rewarded later, he said, because "usually the man in the hospital will have more practice and keep on getting a better one in the end."

As early as 1899, when he was professor of medicine at the University of Michigan, Dock had been a pioneer in instituting the clinical clerkship. His teaching exercises were preserved by the university as the "Clinical Notebooks of George Dock, 1899-1908," which indicate that students at Michigan were given responsibility for patient care. Dock would tell the students that "the patient is under your care as part of your duties" and to "follow up the case as long as the patient is in the hospital, seeing the patient at least once or twice a day."

In 1919, fresh from his triumphs on the Empyema Commission, Dr. Evarts A. Graham, at age 36, was appointed the first full-time professor of surgery and chairman of the department at Washington University School of Medicine. He was only the second full-time professor of surgery in the entire United States; the first was William S. Halsted, who had accepted the full-time chair in surgery at Johns Hopkins five years earlier. The dean of the medical school, Dr. Philip Schaffer, along with medical faculty members G. Canby Robinson and Eugene Opie, had gone to Camp Sheridan near Chicago in May to persuade Graham to take the job.

When he got to the medical school in September of 1919, Graham found only 97 patients at Barnes Hospital, the main teaching hospital for the newly reorganized school, and he began a campaign to convince the medical profession around St. Louis to send more patients there. Over the next 32 years, he developed a strong department with high standards and became one of the most influential surgeons of his time.

The medical school at Washington University had been a proprietary institution (owned and operated by the faculty and dependent on student fees for income) prior to 1906, when Robert S. Brookings, who had become president of the university in 1905, succeeded in making the university assume control of and take financial responsibility for the medical school. From the very beginning in 1891, when an independent institution named the St. Louis Medical College became the Washington University Medical College, the school had distinguished itself among the 30-odd other schools that had played their hour upon the stage during the first 100 years of Missouri medicine. The university added new courses, expanded the faculty and constructed new laboratories for the basic science courses after it took over the medical school.

Despite these improvements, when Abraham Flexner visited the school in 1909, he found it "a little better than the worst I had seen elsewhere, but absolutely inadequate in every essential respect." However, President Brookings was negotiating for the use of Barnes Hospital and St. Louis Children's at the time, and Flexner saw promise in that affiliation.

"There is abundant evidence to indicate that those interested in Washington University appreciate its 'manifest destiny'; it bids fair shortly to possess faculty, laboratories, and hospitals conforming in every respect to ideal standards."

In the reform era that followed Flexner's report, philanthropic foundations made more money available to medical education, and so in January of 1914, Brookings applied for and received a $750,000 grant from the General Education Board, a philanthropic foundation organized in 1902 by John D. Rockefeller, to establish full-time clinical departments. The grant was increased to $1 million in 1916 and local donors added an additional $500,000 to create a $1.5 million nest egg for full-time professorships in medicine, surgery and pediatrics. George Dock accepted the position in medicine, Evarts Graham in surgery and William McKim Marriott in pediatrics. All three established high traditions in clinical medicine and teaching.

In 1912, Flexner had joined the staff of the General Education Board and persuaded Rockefeller to earmark $50 million to implement his recommendations for improving medical education, particularly the establishment of a full-time clinical faculty. The foundation would award grants totaling more than $90 million until 1936; about half of that money went to five medical schools alone—Cornell, the University of Chicago, Johns Hopkins, Vanderbilt and Washington University. (Harvard and Columbia refused to accept the full-time plan—and the foundation's money—but Harvard came up with an alternative, called the geographic full-time plan, that quickly spread to other medical schools. Under this plan, the faculty physician could see private patients but did so in the hospital where he taught).

Washington University stuck with Flexner's full-time plan, under which the professor received a salary only, and benefited greatly from the millions that the General Education Board lavished on the school. With foundation support and a superb full-time clinical faculty in place, President Brookings, a self-educated St. Louis businessman who had made a fortune in merchandising woodenware and was inspired by his long-time friend Andrew Carnegie, turned Washington University into one of the leading medical schools of the era.

"I had heard about Dr. Graham before I met him," Dr. Cole recalled in 1989. "He was known for his research work when he was appointed to the Empyema Commission by the Surgeon General. At that time, during the flu epidemic, a lot of people were getting empyema and surgeons were operating on them the next day after they discovered the infection. As a result, most of those patients died because the mediastinum, the thin wall separating the two cavities surrounding the lungs, needed to be immobilized for a time before operative drainage of one of the cavities. The commission advised that surgery be postponed for several days and the pleural space aspirated before drainage in order to sterilize it. As a result, the mortality rate changed tremendously, from 30 percent to 4 percent. The dean of the medical school was a biochemist and a very smart man. He realized that this man [Graham] had done research to change the mortality rate. On that basis, he appointed Graham head of surgery."

Dr. Cole's clinical years of medical school were filled with long hours, hard study and an incredible volume of information to be absorbed. The curriculum was based on the assumption that after graduation and a year or two of internship, the young physician would be prepared to enter general practice with enough knowledge to deal with almost any medical problem, including most illnesses that needed major surgery. It was not until after World War I that medical schools began to recognize the need for specialization in medical education because of the volume of material that needed to be covered.

What students learned was very much a reflection of the diseases that were prevalent in the hospitals where they studied. From 1918 on through the 1920s, patients suffering from infectious diseases occupied a large percentage of hospital beds. Mortality from pneumonia was high, as was the incidence of tuberculosis. Heroic measures were used to treat TB, such as collapsing the infected lung by injecting air into the pleural cavity or by removing ribs. Diphtheria, scarlet fever and congenital syphilis were also common problems. Infants emaciated from diarrhea due to dietary deficiencies filled the children's wards.

The primitive drug therapy available consisted of such things as Fowler's solution (a compound of arsenic), strychnine and potassium iodide. It wasn't until the 1930s that drug research began producing the first modern drugs, even though Ehrlich's discovery of a compound of arsenic as a treatment for syphilis appeared promising in 1909. Most of the chemicals used to kill microorganisms were extremely toxic to human beings. Some biological serums were available at the time, such as diphtheria antitoxin, which was developed in 1894, but most were so harmful to the patient that proper diagnosis of the infection and scrupulous use of these substances were crucial. Chest surgery was usually done for patients with chronic infections, such as empyema, bronchiectasis (dilatation of small bronchial tubes) and tuberculosis.

The buildup of the clinical departments in medical schools and the new emphasis on research helped to change medical treatment dramatically over the next decades. Warren Cole attended medical school during this transition period and was infused with the ideal of teaching and research that filled the academic air at Washington University School of Medicine just after the first world war. He was a product of the newly arrived clinical scientists who were at the vanguard of an unprecedented explosion in medical discovery and the vast improvement in medical care that continues today. His professors were among the best clinical minds of the time and they taught him the importance of the inquiring medical mind. Before long, Warren Cole was to show his own genius for research.

CHAPTER 6

❧

THE VERY MODEL OF
MEDICAL TRAINING

F lexner's model for the ideal medical school was the Johns Hopkins University School of Medicine in Baltimore. In the reform era that followed the Flexner report, the medical school at Johns Hopkins became the single most significant institution in the spread of scientific medical education in America. Not only was it the prototype by which all others were judged, but many of its graduates disseminated its tenets of education when they became professors at medical schools all around the country.

Washington University was one of the first schools to reflect the Hopkins influence. Washington University president Robert Brookings stated that his intention when the university took over the medical school in 1906 was to "Johns Hopkinize" it. Two of the department heads of the newly revamped school of medicine were Hopkins graduates—Eugene Opie in pathology and Joseph Erlanger in physiology—and the junior faculty they brought in numbered among them Hopkins grads and former residents as well. George Canby Robinson, for example, a 1903 graduate of Johns Hopkins Medical School, went to Washington University in 1913 as associate professor of medicine.

Robinson was responsible for organizing both the outpatient department and the inpatient medical service at

Barnes Hospital, the university's teaching facility. He was so successful at setting up those services that in 1920, using the experience he gained at Washington University, he became dean of the newly formed medical school at Vanderbilt University in Nashville. But before he left, he helped Warren Cole, now with an M.D. degree, secure an internship in medicine at Baltimore City Hospitals under Thomas J. Boggs, whom Robinson knew from medical school and who in 1920 was associate professor of clinical medicine at Hopkins and physician in charge of Baltimore City Hospitals.

Finding an internship at one of the top hospitals in the country was a highly competitive business, but Dr. Robinson made it easy for Warren Cole. "One of my teachers, Canby Robinson, said, 'Have you got an internship? I have a friend in Baltimore who could use someone,'" Dr. Cole said. "Early in my medical school days, I had decided to take up surgery as a specialty, but chose first to take a year of internal medicine to give me a better foundation."

And so young Dr. Cole spent his first year out of medical school, 1920 to 1921, as an intern in internal medicine under Dr. Thomas Boggs at City Hospitals in Baltimore.

The internship in American medical education has its roots in the "house pupil" system that first emerged in the 1820s and 1830s and slowly grew more and more popular. At that time, a handful of students, who were usually chosen by competitive examination either before or after receiving an M.D. degree, resided in a hospital and had some responsibility for patient care, much as house officers do today. After 1850 and the introduction of anesthesia, the role of the house pupil became much more demanding because of the increasing amount of surgery performed in hospitals. Even then, house pupils were overworked and overstressed. The system lasted until 1970 when the separate internship was absorbed into residency training. But until 1970, many graduates of medical schools first took an internship in general medicine and then a residency in a medical or surgical specialty.

The intern was given routine responsibilities that could not be delegated to a student clinical clerk—admission histories, physical examinations, diagnostic procedures, injections and laboratory studies. The year was designed to provide gradually increasing responsibility for patient care, supplemented by formal teaching through hospital rounds and seminars, although the formal instruction was usually casual and unsystematic. Interns treated patients with minor illnesses and injuries in emergency rooms, but generally their time was spent in more routine tasks.

Their hours were long and their pay short. Being on duty for 36 hours at a stretch with little or no sleep was considered one of the initiation rites to becoming a physician, and that system is only today being questioned as a danger to patient care. In 1920, Dr. Cole received $100 a month as an intern at City Hospitals and lived in a building set aside for house staff (interns and residents). At the time, marriage was frowned upon and considered a detriment to the young physician's career.

Internships could be taken in either a teaching hospital or a community hospital. Although the teaching hospitals offered the more academic atmosphere, they served patients who were primarily poor and seriously ill, and often most of the teaching was done by residents who were steeped in new forms of therapy and the diagnosis of exotic illnesses. Community hospitals offered the intern exposure to more common illnesses and patients with a greater variety of social and economic backgrounds, but the teaching staff was comprised of busy private practitioners who had less interest in medical education. Young medical graduates who wanted a career in academic medicine sought an internship in a teaching hospital on a straight service, that is, they trained in one specialty throughout the year rather than rotating through other specialty services. The choices for straight internships in Dr. Cole's day were in internal medicine, surgery or obstetrics.

The institution that became Baltimore City Hospitals, now called Francis Scott Key Medical Center, was established under the name Bay View Asylum in 1866 by the City of Baltimore as an asylum for mental patients and patients with chronic diseases. In 1910, it was substantially enlarged to provide medical and surgical care for Baltimore's indigent citizens. In that same year, while new facilities were being built, the Board of Supervisors of City Charities changed the asylum's name to Baltimore City Hospitals and asked the deans of the four medical schools then operating in Baltimore to nominate candidates to fill the newly created posts of physician-in-chief, surgeon-in-chief and pathologist-in-chief. This pattern of staffing continued until about 1985 when the City Hospitals, drowning in $8 million of debt, were taken over by Johns Hopkins completely.

In 1911, Thomas R. Boggs became physician-in-chief, Arthur M. Shipley surgeon-in-chief, and Milton C. Winternitz pathologist-in-chief. Boggs and Winternitz were from the Hopkins faculty, and Shipley was a rising young man on the faculty of the University of Maryland Medical School. Born in Memphis in 1875, Boggs earned his undergraduate degree at the University of Georgia, where his father was chancellor. He studied medicine for a year at the University of Pennsylvania, then transferred to Johns Hopkins Medical School and graduated in 1901. Thereafter, he spent his entire professional career associated with Hopkins—first as part of the residency staff, then as a part-time professor of clinical medicine. He was known as a scholarly man, modest and retiring, and he was highly respected as a clinician.

"Boggs was one of the key people on the Hopkins faculty," Dr. Cole said. "He was a very fine person and a very knowledgeable man. I felt that an internship in medicine would be helpful to me because there are many things about the workup of a patient that go beyond the scope of a surgeon. That knowledge put me ahead of my competitors when I went to seek a residency in surgery later on."

At the time of his death in 1938, the *Bulletin of the Johns Hopkins Hospital* characterized Dr. Boggs as "a skillful, thorough physician whose attitude towards his patients of every class alike was one of warm sympathetic understanding; a stimulating teacher whose quality of mind, lucidity of expression and ability tellingly to present a subject made what he taught difficult to forget. If a teacher's quality can be measured by his generosity to his colleagues and to his students, his was of the best."

Boggs was particularly interested in training house staff and students. Characteristic of his attitude toward teaching was his book plate, which had a drawing on it of an old ox and a young ox pulling a plow together. Above the drawing was the legend: *A bove majore discit arrare minor*—The young ox learns to plough a straight furrow by working beside an old ox.

According to a story told by J.M.T. Finney, an outstanding surgeon on the part-time staff at Hopkins and one of the founders of the American College of Surgeons, late in 1905, Dr. William Osler, the lion of the original Hopkins medical staff, was making his last ward rounds at the Johns Hopkins Hospital before departing for England to become Regius Professor of Medicine at Oxford University. After he had seen the last patient, Osler handed his stethoscope to a young resident accompanying him on rounds and said, "Now carry on my work." The young man was Dr. Thomas Boggs. As physician-in-chief of Baltimore City Hospitals, Boggs developed a public hospital modeled on the best Oslerian standards of the Johns Hopkins Hospital that provided excellent care to the indigent sick of Baltimore and high-quality instruction to the house staff and medical students.

Public hospitals had their roots in the poor houses developed in colonial days. In America, the sick poor were cared for under a system inherited from English law, which was formulated as the Elizabethan Poor Law of 1601. The law had origins in medieval Italian parishes from the 6th century where tithes were collected by the parish church and used to take care of orphans and the infirm. From the beginning in the United States, poor houses, or almshouses, provided a doctor to care for the sick who were housed in an infirmary. Until the Great Depression of the 1930s, public care for the poor was financed by local contributions and local taxes. It took that jarring social upheaval to bring the federal government into the role of helping to support institutions for the public welfare.

The medical and surgical wards at Baltimore City Hospitals opened in 1911 in a acute care hospital built in the shape of a Y on the banks of Chesapeake Bay. The southwest wing on the first floor of the Y contained the surgical suite, while the southeast wing was taken up with clinical laboratories. But despite the addition of a new building to the hospital complex, chronic problems of insufficient space for patients plagued the institution. The three hospitals that made up the complex were now crowded with both insane patients and acute care patients.

Public acceptance of hospitals as places to get well rather than places to die grew after scientists discovered the role of bacteria in disease, infection and death. Diagnostic techniques and equipment also gave a boost to the image and role of the hospital in health care. First came the discovery of x-rays, which was quickly followed by the refinement of techniques to measure blood pressure and basal metabolism as well as various tests to determine how efficiently body organs were functioning. Some of the procedures could be applied at home, but many required heavy equipment or expensive clinical laboratories only available in hospitals. As a result, more and more illnesses of a medical nature, rather than a surgical one, demanded the facilities of a hospital for proper care.

Boggs was trained by William Osler, who perhaps more than any other physician had a lasting effect on medical education and medical practice in the United States. Osler was both professor of medicine at the Johns Hopkins School of Medicine and physician-in-chief at Johns Hopkins Hospital, and it was on his model that Boggs based the medical service at Baltimore City Hospitals. A consummate clinician, Osler had been born and educated in Canada and so he brought the English tradition of clinical medicine to Hopkins, although he frequently lauded the German accomplishments in medical teaching and research. Osler was among the first to draw on clinical laboratories to aid him in diagnosing illnesses. His strength was in studying and teaching the natural history of disease in hospitalized patients; he was always at his best as a clinical diagnostician. His textbook, *Principles and Practice of Medicine,* became a classic for medical students and practicing physicians.

Training in the seat of the best medical educational institution in the country at that time was invaluable experience for the young Dr. Warren Cole, who would later be charged with developing his own clinical teaching program at the University of Illinois. Osler directly influenced Boggs and Boggs directly influenced Cole who, in turn, directly influenced many others. Each passed along the best traditions of clinical medicine and clinical research, traditions that have led to the explosion of medical innovations available today and have made American medicine and American medical education second to none in the world. Cole was fortunate in having such a wise old ox from which to learn how to plow a straight furrow.

But even after World War I, when more and more patients were going to hospitals for non-surgical care, surgery was what filled many of the hospital beds. Lister had introduced antisepsis as a method of killing germs that could cause infection in surgical patients. After the 1880s, however, asepsis began to displace antisepsis as a method of controlling infection. Asepsis was designed to prevent bacterial contamination of wounds from taking place rather than killing bacteria after contamination.

The earliest aseptic techniques consisted of steam sterilization of surgical dressings and the gowns that surgeons and nurses used in the operating room; thorough cleansing of the surgeons' hands and arms by scrubbing with soap and water, then soaking them in a solution of bichloride of mercury; cleansing and sterilizing the patient's skin at the site of the incision; sterilizing instruments in boiling water and antiseptic solutions; and covering the heads and faces of members of the surgical team with sterile caps and masks.

The first full-time professor of surgery at Johns Hopkins, William Halsted, whom Dr. Cole later called one of the "five pillars of modern surgery," introduced a crucial aspect of aseptic technique in 1889—the use of sterile rubber gloves. Halsted actually thought of using the gloves initially to help protect the hands of his head operating-room nurse, who later became his wife. Her hands were sensitive to bichloride of mercury. One of his residents continued to use the gloves and showed their effectiveness in preventing infection. Halsted made a number of other important discoveries that enhanced the development of surgery. He proved that rough handling of body tissue either by the surgeon's hands or with instruments resulted in poor healing and invited infection. He discovered that silk was a far better suture material than the catgut then in use because it caused less irritation to tissue. And he learned to close surgical incisions layer by layer without tension in order to enhance the healing process.

Halsted's landmark contributions to surgery affected almost every aspect of surgical practice. He pioneered advances in the diagnosis and treatment of thyroid disease, invented an artery clamp that controlled hemorrhage and lessened tissue damage, and devised a special suture for joining surfaces of the intestine. Halsted revolutionized the practice of surgery with an innovative operation for hernia repair and the radical mastectomy to treat breast cancer, which until fairly recent times was considered the operation of choice for that disease.

His meticulously devised surgical techniques were all based on scientific evidence, and they made the craft of surgery a much safer form of medical practice. Halsted's insights into the careful handling of tissue took surgery out of the primitive era of quick and sometimes brutal cutting into an epoch of therapeutic operations that have become more and more daring with each new generation. He led the way to scientific surgery based on solid clinical research and permanently altered man's ability to conquer disease. In his hands, the field of surgery became a true specialty in medicine, rather than something every physician was required to know a little bit about.

Among Halsted's important contributions to medicine was the residency training system he developed. He selected only the best students for his program and trained them to be top surgeons and distinguished teachers. One of Halsted's residents at Hopkins, Harvey Cushing, went on to develop brain surgery as a specialty and made such far-reaching discoveries as the relationship of blood pressure to the patient's condition during surgery and how to treat pituitary tumors by operation.

After his year as a medical intern at Baltimore City Hospitals and his exposure to the most advanced medical and surgical practice available in the country, Warren Cole was anxious to begin his residency in surgery, which, under Halsted's leadership, was emerging as an exciting specialty with the promise of making tremendous strides toward alleviating many of the causes of disease and death that plagued mankind. But Halsted, like many of the pioneers of scientific medicine in America, was at the end of his career in 1921. He died in 1922 of biliary disease at the age of 70.

Dr. Cole decided he wanted to return to Washington University and study surgery in the program run by Evarts Graham. "I almost stayed in the East for my surgical training, but I had heard that Dr. Graham had a great future and was able to inspire the young people under him," Warren recalled many years later. "I wrote to Dr. Graham to ask him for an internship in surgery and fortunately was accepted. I applied for an internship rather than a residency position because I thought that the transition from an internship in another specialty to an assistant residency in surgery was too big a jump. My experience over the next year proved my assumption to be correct. I did a good job in my surgical internship because of the year of medicine I had in back of me. I knew a lot about the diagnosis of illnesses that none of the other students had heard of. And I could diagnose and work up surgical patients well because I had been doing it for a year.

"When the time came, I asked Dr. Graham if I could get an assistant residency under him the next year. Much to my disappointment he said, 'No, I'm sorry, you can't. All the residency positions are taken.' But one of my classmates on the house staff had gone from an internship in internal medicine directly into an assistant residency in surgery the same year that I was a surgical intern. He did a poor job of it because he couldn't manage patients with that degree of responsibility. He made such a bad impression that he was fired at the end of the year, and I was appointed to take his place the next year. I got the residency position because of the training in medicine I had."

Back in St. Louis with a residency appointment assured, Dr. Cole settled into his quarters at Barnes Hospital and looked forward to a three-year residency under Dr. Graham, who was to become Cole's major role model in medicine and what historian Peter Olch called a "pivotal figure in American surgery."

Ironically Dr. Cole began to receive a salary as a resident in surgery of $25 a month, down from the $100 a month he received as an intern at Baltimore City Hospitals but up from the zero salary he got as a surgical intern at Washington University. Under the reasoning of the time, the more desirable the position, the less it paid. Competition for surgical residency slots at the top medical schools was cutthroat and the schools knew they did not have to offer a large salary to attract good people. Dr. Cole accepted the residency and the salary, and gladly, and continued an association with Washington University that was to last until 1936.

CHAPTER 7

FROM STUDENT TO
RESEARCH SCIENTIST

I f the competition to get a residency position was cut-throat, the competition to stay in one was even more so. Prior to World War II, residency staffs were set up along a pyramidal system. At the bottom of the pyramid were the interns. On most services there were two to three times as many interns as first-year residents, twice as many first-year residents as second-year residents and so on up the line until only one survivor remained, like King Kong at the top of the Empire State Building, to become chief resident...the king of the hill. Along the way perfectly capable physicians were drummed out of the system and forced to find another specialty or another position.

Residents lived in the hospital because room and board represented a major part of their compensation. Being married was verboten. In his retirement years, Dr. Cole wrote a humorous anecdote that underlines the intensity of the competition for a residency position:

"Unaware of his possible influence on my career, Dr. Vilray Blair (a famous plastic surgeon) asked me one day during my surgical internship to go with him to make rounds on his patients at St. Luke's Hospital, after he finished at Barnes Hospital. Sometime later, I learned that Dr. Blair was thinking of asking me to join his plastic group after I finished my training, and he wanted to get acquainted with me. It happened that I had promised to go out on a blind date with a nurse from Barnes Hospital that night, along with several other couples from the hospital. We were going to take a cruise on the River Queen, a fancy river boat that plies the Mississippi River out of St. Louis.

"We were set to meet at the dock from which the boat left at 7:30 that evening. I assumed that Dr. Blair would complete his rounds long before that time. But Dr. Blair had a huge practice and he was delayed at Barnes. On our way to St. Luke's Hospital from Barnes, we passed a snack bar and he said, 'We'd better stop here for a sandwich.' All of this consumed a lot of time and I was beginning to worry about my date on the River Queen. I was a very modest fellow in my intern days and I was afraid to say anything to Dr. Blair.

"I was also afraid to let Dr. Blair know that I was going out with the nurse, lest he tell Dr. Graham who was soon to make appointments to his residency staff, an appointment I was seeking most emphatically. There were no married residents at that time. It was known that Dr. Barney Brooks on Dr. Graham's staff had made a statement that if he were the boss, a resident would be fired if he got married. We learned later that Dr. Graham probably was not so strict, but I did not want to take any chances; I wanted the residency so badly.

"Soon it became apparent that if I wanted to keep my date, I would have to leave Dr. Blair to finish his rounds alone. I decided to take no chances, and so I continued with Dr. Blair past the time I was supposed to meet the crowd at the River Queen dock. The next day, naturally, I apologized very profusely to the older nurse who had arranged the blind date for me.

"A short time later, I actually met the young nurse who was going to be my blind date. She was a very charming girl and I fell madly in love with her. I tried to get a date with her but she declined two or three attempts. She was so attractive, I realized, that I would probably have asked her to marry me if we had spent time together. And, if we had been married, we probably would have had children, thus making it essential that I stop my residency training and go into private practice. This would have destroyed my surgical career. So

Dr. Blair unknowingly took a role in shaping my career and my life."

Dr. Leon Bromberg, a lifelong friend of Dr. Cole who was a resident in internal medicine at Washington University at the same time that Cole was there, recalled years later Cole's effect on women. "Warren, virile and wiry though he is, has always been of a thin build—with a hungry look. I confess this was the source of envy from other interns and youthful associates for it was one of the factors that made all of the beautiful nurses want to mother him. Naturally, they all admired his quiet competence and gentle nature with patients and students too, and his shyness with women also seemed to add a magnetic quality."

When Warren Cole was a first-year resident at Washington University School of Medicine in 1922, there were six first-year residents, three second-year residents, and one senior resident. Presiding over all the surgical interns and residents was Evarts Ambrose Graham, the first full-time professor of surgery at the school, a man dedicated to the idea of teaching and research as ways to elevate the standards of surgical education and surgical practice. It did not take much intelligence for the house staff to figure out that the way to Graham's heart and the chief resident's position was through research.

"Dr. Graham was strong for research," Dr. Cole said. "All of his lectures were based on research. He was strongly interested in the research phase of medicine, and he always had us working on some research project, no matter what else was going on. When I was in medical school at Washington University, I was in Barnes Hospital most of the time and I seldom got across the street to where the research labs were. But later on, when I was a resident, I shared an office in the department of surgery next to the research labs and I began to get interested in research there. We were invited to do research in the animal labs that the department of surgery maintained. Practically all of the members of the department were doing research at that time."

Surprisingly, Evarts Graham himself never went through a conventional residency program, but he did spend seven years researching the chemical aspects of medical problems following an internship. Born in Chicago in 1883, Graham was the son of a surgeon associated with Rush Medical College and Presbyterian Hospital in that city. After graduating from Princeton in 1904, he returned to his home town for medical school at the University of Chicago. His chemistry and biology credits from Princeton allowed him to complete the first two years of medical school in one year, and he spent the next two years in clinical training at Rush Medical College, the clinical arm of the University of Chicago. After he received his M.D. degree in 1907, he interned for a year at Presbyterian Hospital, then worked as a fellow in pathology at Rush and a special student in chemistry at the University of Chicago.

Graham spent the next seven years in laboratory research. During this time, he was also an assistant and later an instructor in surgery at Rush Medical College and assistant surgeon and then assistant attending surgeon at Presbyterian Hospital (1909-1915). No one knows for sure how much actual surgery Graham performed in this period of his professional life, but all indications are that most of his time was taken up with research into the physiology and chemistry of the human disease process and very little with operative surgery.

However, in 1915, he forsook both academic medicine and research and headed for small town practice in Mason City, Iowa. Here he became familiar with the life of a practicing surgeon and gained practical experience in operative surgery. But he encountered a problem for which his expertise in research had not prepared him. The issue was fee-splitting, the practice, then pervasive, by which a surgeon would kick back a part of his fee to the physician who referred the patient to him. "Dr. Graham had ideas of his own about how a surgeon should live," Dr. Cole recalled. "He was vitally opposed to fee-splitting. The fee-splitters drove him out of his practice of surgery in his little town in Iowa. He was opposed to them and would not live with them." In fact, Graham launched a public campaign in Mason City against fee-splitting and another evil of the time, ghost surgery—surgery done by someone unknown to the patient. He made public pronouncements against the practices and generated newspaper publicity. His local colleagues were infuriated, but he stuck to his principles.

Graham continued throughout his life to be a firebrand in the fight to elevate the standards of surgery and surgeons. In 1935, he was appointed by the American Surgical Association as chairman of a Committee on the Elevation of Surgical Standards, a forerunner of the American Board of Surgery, an organization that certifies to the public, through written and oral examinations, that a surgeon is properly qualified to do surgery. He further crusaded to improve surgery by becoming involved with the American College of Surgeons, first as president and later as chairman of the board of regents.

"He was my role model in surgery," Dr. Cole said. "He was a very independent individual, stern, and quite a disciplinarian. Many considered him someone who was not easy to get along with. But he was always good to me. He never spoke a cross word to me in his life."

As was the case in internal medicine, the training that Warren Cole received as a surgical resident was very much dependent upon the surgical diseases prevalent at the time. As Evarts Graham demonstrated while he was on the Empyema Commission, once surgeons solved the problem of negative pressure in the chest region, they were able to perform chest surgery routinely for such chronic infections as empyema, bronchiectasis (dilatation of small bronchial tubes) and tuberculosis. Graham eventually opened up the entire field of thoracic surgery when he performed the first successful removal of an entire lung in 1933. After that, surgeons began to operate more and more on patients with cancer and other tumors of the lungs, but those kinds of operations were not possible when Cole was a resident.

Owen Wangensteen, who was a great teacher of surgery in his own right at the University of Minnesota, described the times in this way: "The medical student attending surgical wards today is confronted with a sight quite different than that of the intern days in 1920-1921. More than one-third of the patients admitted to Gillette Hospital in St. Paul then came because of tuberculosis of lymph nodes and bones. Today none are to be seen there. A decade later, one of the important activities of our Surgical Service was treatment of pulmonary [tuberculosis by] excision. These, too, have disappeared."

According to most accounts, Graham was not a technically gifted surgeon. The English surgeon Lord Brock, who studied under Graham for a year in 1930 to 1931, observed, "Graham was in the very front rank of surgeons, but not as an operator. In his best years I judged him as rather heavy-handed and lacking in practical flair. When I saw him in later years, I found him a very poor operator. I thought how remarkable it was that such a great surgeon who had made great contributions to surgery could be such an indifferent practical performer."

But what Graham lacked in technical proficiency he more than made up for in his ability to train and influence a generation of general and thoracic surgeons in the best aspects of scientific surgery based on solid research. He was also a powerhouse on the executive staff of the medical school because of his outspoken nature and strong stand on ethical issues. Dr. Barry Wood, a former colleague on the medical faculty at Washington University, said of Graham at a memorial service for him, "Unlike so many departmental chairmen, his primary concern was always for the medical school as a whole rather than for his own department. Although his own department was always the biggest earner, he insisted that a generous portion of the fees earned by his full-time staff be turned over to the medical school rather than revert to the department of surgery. His firm stand on this issue greatly increased the solidarity of the medical faculty."

Medical historian Peter Olch ranks Graham with Halsted and Cushing as part of a troika of the most influential surgeons of this century: "Evarts Ambrose Graham, along with William S. Halsted and Harvey Cushing, profoundly influenced the progress and direction of surgery in this century. Of the three, the breadth of influence is probably greatest for the St. Louis surgeon who steadfastly battled to elevate the standards of surgical education and practice."

From the perspective of hindsight at the end of the 20th century, it is apparent that Warren Cole came to surgery on the wings of some of the eagles of the profession. He looked up to and emulated the men who were to shape the very nature of surgery and the way it was to be practiced throughout the century. He, in turn, was to take a significant role in furthering their aims and extending the role of research in education and surgical care.

Although the residency system had been introduced in the United States in the late 19th century, residencies were available only in the leading hospitals before World War I. But residency programs spread rapidly in the 1920s, especially after the American Medical Association established principles for residencies in 1923. The AMA required residencies of two to three years, although short courses were also permitted. The proliferation of residency programs was a major development in medical education that led to vast improvements in the quality of surgery in the first third of this century. One reason was that it promoted the expansion of clinical research, especially in the leading medical schools. Residents did not have private practices and were able to devote their time to detailed study of their specialty. "Graduate training in surgery," said Frederick A. Coller when he was made president of the American Surgical Association in 1944, "is largely a development since 1920 and has done more to stimulate original scientific work in surgery in this country than has any other force."

Dr. Graham created a heady atmosphere for research at Washington University, and Warren Cole soon caught the fever. Cole immediately showed his genius for recognizing fundamental medical truths by observing simple physical activity. Barely two months after he began his first-year residency under Dr. Graham, in November of 1922, he published his first research paper, "Results of Treatment of Fractured Femurs in Children," in the Archives of Surgery. Cole's study was done under the aegis of Dr. M. B. Clopton, a former resident of Halsted at Johns Hopkins, who was now at St. Louis Children's Hospital. For the study, Dr. Cole reviewed the treatment of fractured thighbones in 35 infants and children and concluded that overhead traction was the best method of treatment among the six that were used: overhead traction, plaster casts, splints, horizontal traction, open reduction and modified Steinman pin.

The conclusion was of value but not earthshaking. However, in the course of the study, Cole painstakingly measured the bones of each little patient. He found that the shortening of the bone, which occurs immediately after fracture because the bone fragments overlap one another, tends to correct itself as the child grows. Nature heals its own.

"Perhaps one of the most striking observations," he wrote in the article, "is the absence of shortening seen in cases which healed with fragments distinctly in an overriding position. Moreover, when the patient returns a few years later, the affected extremity shows no shortening. Repeated roentgenograms of the knee joints a few weeks and a few years after treatment reveal no separation of the femur from the tibia due to stretching of the ligaments about the knee joint. The question arises as to the location of the compensation. The ligaments of the ankle are not included in the traction at all. Furthermore, one cannot conceive of the hip joint allowing much room for lengthening of the extremity. Apparently, the only explanation remaining is that young bone yields to the constant pull, and thus makes up for the few centimeters necessary for compensation."

When Cole first presented his observations to the medical staff at Washington University, Dr. Barney Brooks, another of Halsted's residents who had set up the surgical pathology laboratory at Washington University and pursued research into bone regeneration, was incredulous. "Dr. Brooks very politely said he didn't see how that could happen, that it didn't sound reasonable," Dr. Cole recalled. "He threw cold water on my conclusion. That sort of stopped the discussion and I fell pretty flat. After the meeting, I hurried to get out of there. Dr. Opie came running up behind me, took me by the shoulder and said, 'Dr. Cole, don't take that remark of Dr. Brooks seriously because I think he's wrong and you're right. Study that some more.' Well, naturally, I was very pleased."

Dr. Eugene Opie had reason for defending the young investigator. Opie was a member of the first graduating class of the Johns Hopkins School of Medicine in 1897. While still a medical student, he disproved current assumptions about cells in the pancreas and demonstrated that severe injury to cellular masses in the pancreas (the islets of Langerhans) causes diabetes. This finding later led to the discovery of insulin.

Cole continued his research and in October of 1925 published a follow-up study in the *Annals of Surgery* titled "Compensatory lengthening of the femur in children after fracture." The second study reinforced the validity of his observation that for the majority of children who suffer a fracture of the femur, the thighbone (and the leg bone or tibia) will lengthen as the child grows to compensate for any shortening caused by the fracture. He also found that an operation to set the bone straight (operative reduction) is rarely needed and sometimes results in a deformity of the leg.

In another early study, published in 1924, Cole reviewed the case of a patient who died from systemic blastomycosis, a yeast-like infection that is rare today since the advent of antibiotics. Normally, the disease started with a skin infection and then spread throughout the patient's body. "Although frequent recoveries are encountered among the cases whose disease is limited to the skin, the fatality of systemic infection is almost absolute," Dr. Cole wrote. Cole's study described how the organism showed itself, the course it took and the effectiveness of available treatments.

These studies showed Cole's brilliant use of simple observation in medical research and his ability to analyze what he observed and show its impact on medical care. At 24, he showed tremendous promise, and that kept him in good standing in Dr. Graham's residency pyramid.

One day in early spring of 1923, toward the end of Dr. Cole's first year of residency training, Graham called him to his office to discuss his appointment for the following year. Because all the residents faced the constant threat of being dropped from the program, Cole feared he was going to be fired.

"When I received this call I immediately thought, 'There are my walking papers and I am going to be relegated to the bush leagues somewhere,'" he wrote in 1960. "On my way to Dr. Graham's office, which in those days was across the street from Barnes Hospital, I did a lot of thinking, wishful thinking it was, trying to justify my reappointment to the second-year residency, even though I knew very well that Dr. Graham's mind was no doubt completely made up about my dismissal, and nothing I could say would change it. All of us knew him as a man of firm conviction who stuck tightly to ideas, almost to the point of stubbornness, unless someone presented very good evidence showing he was wrong.

"Nevertheless, as I crossed the street I began assembling data which might be used in my behalf. This wishful thinking built up almost to a point of resentment. After all, had I not worked night and day throughout the several months of my residency, leaving the hospital no more than two or three evenings per month? Also, had I not fulfilled Koch's postulate on the undiagnosed patient with systemic blastomycosis and demonstrated blastomycetes in the lungs of a guinea pig after inoculation of secretions from a patient's skin ulcer? However, by the time I reached his office I was fairly well resigned to my fate.

"Dr. Graham's greeting was unusually friendly and my concern was neutralized, particularly when he said he had a laboratory experiment in mind which he hoped I would be willing to work on full time the following year, beginning July 1. He relieved any remaining apprehension I had by telling me he wanted me to resume my residency the following year."

CHAPTER 8

❧

LANDING A MUSKIE: THE DISCOVERY OF CHOLECYSTOGRAPHY

The reason Evarts Graham was so friendly on that spring day in 1923 and the reason he wanted his star researcher Warren Cole to take time from his residency training and spend a year in the lab was that Graham was on to something important.

In our era of computerized scanning devices and magnetic imaging machines, it is important to remember that for most of the 20th century, x-rays were the only way of visualizing man's internal organs in order to detect the presence of disease. Professor William Conrad Roentgen from Wurzburg, Germany, first reported the discovery of x-rays in 1895. In 1898, Walter B. Cannon, who was then a medical student at Harvard University, found that when he fed a button to a dog, he could watch the button pass down the dog's esophagus and into its stomach with the use of x-rays. Cannon's discovery opened up the whole field of diagnosis of gastrointestinal tract disorders.

But widespread use of x-rays did not come about until World War I when they were used to help diagnose the wounded. It was not until then that many physicians became aware of the value of this diagnostic technique. Even Washington University did not get its first x-ray machine until after the war.

In 1918, one of Halsted's residents at Johns Hopkins, Walter E. Dandy, developed a way to visualize brain tumors on x-ray screens by injecting air into the cavities of the brain. The air bubbles showed up as negative shadows on x-ray pictures and enabled brain surgeons and neurologists to see tumors and other lesions in the brain. In a report published in February of 1923, Earl Osborne and Leonard Rowntree and others revealed they had found that concentrated sodium iodide was opaque to x-rays. When the investigators injected sodium iodide into a vein and took x-rays of the kidney region while the sodium iodide was being concentrated and excreted by the kidneys, they obtained an x-ray image of the kidneys, ureters and urinary bladder.

This and previous research led Graham to believe that a similar substance could be found to help visualize the gallbladder by x-rays. The task that Graham had in mind for Dr. Cole was to try to discover that substance so that physicians could more accurately diagnose human gallbladder disease. Graham was familiar with the work of John Abel and Leonard Rowntree at Johns Hopkins, who in 1909 demonstrated that phenolphthalein compounds are excreted by the liver into the bile and that the compounds remained in the liver for several hours after ingestion. In addition, in 1921, Drs. Rous and McMaster from the Rockefeller Institute had shown that the bile from the liver enters the gallbladder and is concentrated there eightfold to tenfold.

"It was Dr. Graham's idea that if a heavier halogen such as iodine could be attached to the phenolphthalein radical, the bile might be impervious to the x-ray," Dr. Cole wrote in the *American Journal of Surgery* in February 1960. Cole set out to prove Graham's theory.

He first went to a commercial drug company in St. Louis, Mallinckrodt Chemical Works, and requested several halogenated compounds, including tetraiodophenolphthalein and sodium phenoltetrachlorphthalein. He tried the sodium compound first, but the atomic weight of the chlorine it contained was too low to produce an x-ray image. Chlorine has an atomic weight of only 35.5, whereas iodine has an atomic weight of 127. "It was basic information that elements with a high atomic weight would cast a better radiologic shadow than would elements with a low atomic weight," Cole wrote. "Knowing this, we thought it desirable to try strontium and calcium salts of the halogenated phenolphthaleins rather than sodium.

"For several months, one after another, we tried the sodium, calcium and strontium salts of tetrabromphenol-phthalein and tetraiodophenolphthalein, confining the injections to dogs and rabbits." Cole injected about 200 dogs and rabbits, but no gallbladder shadows showed up on the x-rays. The experiments were time-consuming because it took six to ten hours for the gallbladder to concentrate the compounds to the greatest degree. So he injected the animals at eight or nine in the morning and did not take the x-rays until after five.

The discovery of the means to visualize the human gall-bladder was a case of the old dictum that chance favors the prepared mind. After nearly five months of disappointing results, Cole finally saw a gallbladder shadow on the x-ray of one of the dogs. He was reassured by the denseness of the shadow that the result could be duplicated, at least in animals. "As soon as I saw the film I called Dr. Graham, who was working late as usual. We stood there admiring the dripping film with a white blob in the center, as if we had found a treasure chest full of gold. After a few moments of silence he slapped me on the back and announced enthusiastically, 'Well Warren, we have a muskie on the line, and if the line doesn't break or the boat capsize, we should land him.'"

But the muskie turned out to be an elusive catch. Cole injected two or three more dogs with the same compound (calcium tetrabromphenolphthalein) over the next few days but the results were not the same—no shadow appeared on the x-rays. He reviewed the method he used to concoct and inject the compound, but he still could find no reason why in a single case he obtained an excellent shadow of the gall-bladder and not in any others. Finally it occurred to him to ask the lab assistant, or diener as he was called, if he had given any special care to that one dog.

"Bill hesitated, stammered a bit, and finally announced that he could think of no way in which that animal differed from the others," Dr. Cole remembered. "However, his expression of apprehension melted considerably when he learned that that dog was a favored one, and very meekly, as if fearing a sharp reprimand from me, he muttered, 'Well, Dr. Cole, there was one thing somewhat different. I forgot to feed the dog the morning you injected him.'

"I lunged at him, apparently like a wild animal, trying to slap him on the back and grasp his hand in appreciation at the same time. He retreated hastily, no doubt thinking I was going to manhandle him. However, I quickly convinced him I was merely trying to express my appreciation for the great favor he had unknowingly conferred upon me. The lack of food during the test with this dog represented a definite difference from the routine carried out with the other dogs, and I was willing to assume it might be a vital point." Eureka!

Cole, always the compleat researcher, found out that a scientist named E.A. Boyden had reported at the annual meeting of the American Society of Zoologists earlier that year that food triggers the filling and emptying of the gallbladder, at least in cats. Boyden had not, however, figured out the physical mechanics of it all. "Nevertheless, I felt confident," Dr. Cole wrote, "we had now discovered a change in routine which would duplicate the excellent shadow encountered in the animal accidentally having the test made during a starvation period. Subsequent experiments during the next few days proved that the role of food in the prevention of filling of the gallbladder was an all-powerful one."

Now that he knew he could visualize the gallbladder in animals, Cole moved quickly to do the same in human beings. Although he had used a bromine phthalein compound for the animal experiments, he was aware that an iodine phthalein would create a superior x-ray shadow. But the animal experiments revealed an inconsistent record of toxicity with the use of iodine compounds (he later discovered this reaction was due to impurities in the drugs). Furthermore, the lethal dose—or the amount that will cause death—of iodine phthalein was about one-fifth of the dose required for use in humans, whereas the lethal dose of bromine phthalein was a full one-third of the human dose. Thus bromine was safer.

So when Cole chose a compound for his experiments in

humans, he started with the same one he had used in dogs, calcium tetrabromphenolphthalein. "I began the clinical use of the solution very cautiously, giving 1 gram of tetra-bromphenolphthalein to the first patient. I increased the dose for the next four patients by 1 gram each, giving 5 grams to the fifth patient. This patient experienced the first reaction I encountered, nothing more than a short feeling of warmth over the entire body. I gave 6 grams to the sixth patient, again with no more reaction than a slight feeling of warmth. However, at this point I had used up my share of good luck; in the seventh patient tachycardia [quickening of the heart rate], headache, vertigo and nausea developed, as it did in many thereafter. With the small doses used in the first few patients, we did not expect to obtain visualization of the gall-bladder; we were merely testing the drug for toxicity. I had given the material to nine patients before obtaining the slight-est evidence of a shadow."

This slight evidence was encouragement enough for Dr. Cole to continue. Then, at last, came the first positive visual-ization ever of a human gallbladder, a phenomenon now known as cholecystography. The patient, a woman who also happened to be a nurse at Barnes Hospital, was the sixteenth person he had injected.

The date was February 21, 1924. At 7:00 am, Cole mixed six grams of tetrabromphenolphthalein with 1.1 grams of cal-cium hydroxide and two grams of calcium lactate in 350 cu-bic centimeters of water. By 9:00 am, he had boiled and then cooled the mixture to sterilize it and was ready to inject it. The lesson learned from the fasting dog was not forgotten, and so the woman took the test without breakfast.

"I had already learned that rapid injection of this solu-tion tended to increase the reaction. Accordingly, I gave the injection very slowly, hoping to avoid a reaction completely. However, my hopes were blasted. After injection of slightly over half of the solution the patient began complaining of nausea, followed shortly by pain in the back and elsewhere. I stopped the injection and waited ten minutes; the nausea dis-appeared, so I renewed the injection. After I injected 40 cc. more, the patient's nausea returned, so I stopped the injection again for a few minutes.

"After repeating the process of stopping and starting the injection several times, I was finally able to complete injection of the entire amount, although it required over an hour for completion. I had been watching her pulse and blood pressure closely, and since they had remained practically normal, I had the courage to proceed with the injection until I had injected all of the solution. It is fortunate that we obtained a good visualization of the gallbladder; otherwise, after seeing the patient in such misery with severe nausea, retching and in generalized pain, I doubt that I would have had the courage or cruelty to continue injecting other patients."

The patient was being examined for pain in the area of the kidneys and gallbladder. Cole knew enough about the physiology of the gallbladder to realize that clear visualization on x-ray plates could only be gotten with a non-diseased gallbladder. And so he could eliminate gallbladder disease as a possible diagnosis for the woman, and he saved her—and countless others in future years—a needless gallbladder operation. This first clear shadow convinced Graham and Cole that their theory was right and spurred them to continue testing it.

Their first task was to refine the solution so that it would not cause the severe side effects. In an effort to reduce negative reactions to the mixture, Cole substituted sodium for calcium as the alkali needed to dissolve the otherwise insoluble phenolphthalein. He then conducted a series of tests on dogs to discover exactly what reactions various foods and chemicals caused. "After much experimentation, I learned that the sphincteric action of the sphincter of Oddi could be controlled by acid and alkali. By cannulating [inserting a tube into] the common [bile] duct and connecting the tube to a manometer system, I learned that substituting 75 to 150 cc. of 0.5 per cent sodium hydroxide for saline in the stomach caused the pressure to rise 100 to 225 mm.Hg. Replacement of the sodium hydroxide with 75 to 150 cc. of 0.5 per cent hydrochloric acid caused an immediate drop in pressure of 75 to 150 mm.Hg., indicating that the acid caused a relaxation of the sphincter and alkali caused a contraction. As a consequence of this experiment, we advised and continued the use of 2.5 gm. of sodium bicarbonate every three hours while the patient was awake, during the first 24 to 48 hours following injection."

Shortly after they began using sodium in the solution, they substituted iodine for bromine because the higher atomic weight of the iodine allowed for smaller, and safer, doses (3.5 grams for an adult). They next tried giving the resultant mixture, sodium tetraiodophenolphthalein, orally. Although intravenous injections proved to yield clearer shadows, oral administration of the solution avoided most of the serious physical reactions. However, nausea, vomiting and diarrhea were common with the oral method. Cole and Graham continued to experiment with IV injections for several years, and they found that they could administer less (2.5 grams) and still get clear x-ray shadows of normal gallbladders. Other clinicians who subsequently used the test—which came to be called the Graham-Cole test—gave the solution orally.

"We found out early," Cole wrote, "that the drug reactions were due to the phenolphthalein radical and were not related to the bromine or iodine or base used to dissolve the acid powder. The amazing feature about these reactions, which is still difficult to understand, is that in spite of their severity and frequency, fatalities were practically nonexistent. Of the 2,000 or 3,000 patients to whom we gave the drugs orally or intravenously, there was only one death, and it could not be classified as a direct fatality resulting from cholecystography. The patient, a woman about 68 years old, had a fairly severe reaction consisting of nausea, vomiting, vertigo and chill and died of vascular collapse during the night about 20 hours later. We did not obtain an autopsy on this patient, but since the vascular collapse occurred 15 hours after the injection (of sodium tetrabromphenolphthalein), it seems likely that she had a coronary occlusion or perhaps a pulmonary embolus."

The reactions were classified into first- and second-degree reactions. First-degree reactions included vertigo, headache, backache, slight nausea, weakness and rash, while second-degree reactions were severe nausea, vomiting, chill, circulatory depression, fever and severe stomach cramps. Patients usually recovered from their reactions within four or five hours after an injection. As Cole continued his testing, he was able to obtain purer ingredients for his solution, and that alone decreased the incidence and frequency of reactions from both oral and intravenous administration.

Once they had gotten a handle on how to minimize drug reactions, Cole and Graham turned their attention to interpreting the shadows. They asked Dr. Sherwood Moore, who was then head of the department of radiology at Washington University School of Medicine, to join the research. With Moore's help, they found that if the patient's gallbladder was healthy, a shadow would begin to appear on x-ray films about four hours after IV administration, and it would reach maximum density about 12 hours after the patient was injected; but in another 12 hours the shadow would be just about gone. If the drug was given orally, the shadow appeared in nine or ten hours and reached maximum density in 18 or 20 hours.

"The mechanism of emptying of the gallbladder was obviously of great importance in the interpretation of the variations in the density of the shadow. It was known that the normal gallbladder wall could absorb large quantities of water, but it was questionable whether it could absorb the halogenated phenolphthaleins. [Glover] Copher, who began working with Dr. Graham and myself at about the same time Sherwood Moore did, conducted an experiment to see if this were true. He produced dense shadows of the gallbladder with sodium tetraiodophenolphthalein and then ligated the common duct. The shadows persisted for days with very little change, indicating that the opaque media left the gallbladder as it entered, by way of the cystic and common ducts and not by absorption into the lymphatics or blood vessels. The change in the size of the shadow was difficult to explain, but utilizing the knowledge that a fat meal empties the gallbladder, we concluded that this contraction of the shadow was related to the ingestion of food."

The investigators already knew that if a shadow did not appear on the x-rays, the gallbladder was diseased, but they did not know how to interpret a faint shadow. They eventually found out that a slight shadow indicated that the gallbladder was impaired. Both cholesterol and calcium gallstones were apparent on the x-rays as defects on the shadows.

The Graham-Cole test soon spread throughout the world as the best method of diagnosing gallbladder disease and stones in the gallbladder. Ironically, radiologists at first showed some resistance to the test. "We presented cholecystography at various medical meetings," Dr. Cole wrote, "but relied on Dr. Moore to take care of the presentations at the radiological meetings. For some strange reason, cholecystography was received early with much less enthusiasm by our friends in radiology than any other group. About that time, the technic of diagnosing gallbladder disease by variations in the shadow of the diseased gallbladder and by examining the bile obtained by tube from the duodenum was being developed; I do not blame the radiologic profession for being reluctant to have a third method of diagnosing gallbladder disease introduced to add to the confusion and controversy."

Professional resistance did not last long, however. In 1926, the American Roentgen Ray Society awarded Cole and Graham the Leonard Research Prize for developing cholecystography. And a year later, the St. Louis Medical Society gave them a certificate of merit in recognition of their discovery.

For 17 years, Cole's discovery, tetraiodophenolphthalein, remained the drug used by the medical profession to visualize the human gallbladder on x-ray films and to diagnose disease in that organ. In the early 1940s, two other scientists, Dohrn and Diedrich, found a safer contrast agent for cholecystography and medical science moved on. But history will remember Warren Cole as the innovator of the original agent and a pioneer in the field of x-ray technology.

Cholecystography remains as a classic discovery in the history of medicine. From Cole's basic research has evolved the modern method of oral cholecystography, which experts consider one of the most reliable diagnostic procedures available to medicine. It remained the mainstay of gallbladder imaging until the late 1970s when imaging techniques based on sound waves (ultrasonography) dethroned Cole's technique. Over the years, the test has been used primarily to diagnose gallstones. Nearly 20 million people in the United States have these pesky little crystals, and each year more than half a million people are hospitalized for gallstone disease. Despite the advent of newer methods of imaging, two million oral cholecystograms are still taken yearly in this country. Few methods of diagnosing illness have stood the test of time so well.

Tetraiodophenolphthalein remained the drug of choice for the procedure until the discovery of iodoalphionic acid in 1943, which in turn was replaced by iopanoic acid in the early 1950s. Since the 1950s, other imaging agents have been developed, such as calcium and sodium ipodate. The major aim of developing new drugs for cholecystography was to eliminate the risk of side effects for patients, although iopanoic acid has proven over the long term to be relatively nontoxic.

In 1928, Graham, Cole, Copher and Moore published a textbook called *Diseases of the Gallbladder and Bile Ducts*, which climaxed five years of research after that day in 1923 when Evarts Graham called to his office a worried Warren Cole, who thought he was going to be fired.

CHAPTER 9

❧

CERTAIN FEATURES OF EXCELLENCE

N eedless to say, Graham rehired Cole to resume his residency training following the year off to research cholecystography. The Mallinckrodt Chemical Works, which is now a multimillion dollar drug company, took over the manufacture of Cole's iodine compound and poured money into Graham's department for further research into x-ray imaging. Cole himself never received a cent for his discovery.

Graham and Cole and their colleagues continued researching through Cole's remaining residency years and into the years after 1926, when Cole became an instructor in surgery at Washington University School of Medicine. "There were so many ideas related to this research that we stuck with the original idea for five years," Dr. Cole remembered. "We tried to produce a shadow of the pancreas and kidneys and other organs. Those attempts occupied a great deal of our time. We did find some chemicals that produced shadows of the kidneys, but somebody else found a better substance."

Between 1924 and 1928, Graham, Cole and Copher (and sometimes Moore) published 18 articles in various scientific journals about cholecystography and related findings. (Cole subsequently recounted the story of the discovery of cholecystography in medical journals some seven times between 1960 and 1982.) But despite all this concentrated activity, Cole began to diversify his research interests at Washington University, a characteristic that was to become a hallmark of his entire professional career.

In 1927, when he became an instructor in surgery, Dr. Cole published a report in the respected *Annals of Surgery* on how to stitch up heart wounds. Cole reported his experience in treating a taxi driver who had been stabbed in the chest and rushed to St. Louis City Hospital for treatment in 1926. His opening paragraph sounds naive in our era of big city crime and heroic heart transplants, but it reflects the state of cardiac surgery in Cole's residency days when he actually performed the operation:

"Although the suture of wounds of the heart has ceased to be a strictly rare operation, it is sufficiently infrequent to be encountered by the individual surgeon perhaps only once or twice, if at all, in years of experience on an accident service. However, in view of the strict urgency of such operations, every surgeon should be practically as well qualified to handle such cases as he would a patient who needed a tracheotomy. In 1920, Truffier assembled the reports of 305 cases of suture of the heart with a mortality of 49.6 percent. The following case is reported not only because of recovery, but more especially because of the acquisition of complications in rapid succession, with a recovery from each in a manner almost unbelievable."

One of Cole's closest friends, Dr. Leon Bromberg, who was Cole's roommate for eight years while they were both instructors at the university, recalled the incident for a newspaper writer in 1966:

"One of my most vivid and dramatic recollections of Warren Cole as a young resident was when a man was brought into St. Louis City Hospital stabbed in the heart. There he was, apparently moribund, with the knife still in place and moving with each feeble beat of the heart into which it had been plunged. Remember now that this was 41 years ago, long before the heart-lung machines and the trained teams and laboratory and mechanical aids available today. Warren immediately used the sound and steady surgical judgment which has stood him in good stead until today. He did not attempt to pull the knife out; that would have left a gaping, bleeding wound in the ventricle and killed the patient," Dr Bromberg said.

"It was probably his first chest operation on a human being. Certainly it was the first cardiac operation I can recall. Cole opened up the chest as though he had done this all of his life. There wasn't time to call for help from a senior surgeon that night, and it turned out that none was needed. Warren skillfully put a purse-string suture around the pulsating wound in the heart and as he tightened it to control hemorrhage, an assistant slowly withdrew the knife. Dr. Alfred Goldman and others of us who had witnessed this lifesaving procedure (that patient recovered fully) rushed to congratulate Cole and say: 'This is great! We ought to let the *Post-Dispatch* know about it.' But he was the least impressed of all of us with this surgical triumph. He went back to the interns' quarters on the second floor to resume a penny-ante poker game."

The whole field of thoracic surgery, the specialty concerned with the chest region, was one of Graham's great interests. Indeed, he did more than anyone else to open up the field. Graham had received the coveted Samuel D. Gross prize in 1920 for his triumph on the Empyema Commission, one of the most important early contributions to thoracic surgery. "Dr. Graham's work on empyema and cholecystography made him an international figure," notes medical historian Peter Olch. "His interests returned to disorders of the chest, a field in which he became this country's leader. Within a short period, Graham emerged as the most influential person in thoracic surgery."

But Graham's landmark contribution still lay ahead. In 1933, Graham became the first surgeon to successfully remove an entire lung from a person. The patient, a Pittsburgh obstetrician, had lung cancer, and Graham had intended to remove only part of the lung. Once he opened the man's chest, however, he realized that the tumor was so big he would have to take out all of the lung. The obstetrician survived and, ironically, lived to attend a memorial service for Dr. Graham 24 years later. Graham died of lung cancer. In another twist of irony, Graham, a heavy smoker, did some of the initial experiments to show the causal relationship between cigarette smoking and the rapidly rising incidence of cancer of the lung.

At the time of Graham's death in 1957, Dr. Cole wrote about his chief's influence as a teacher for the *Bulletin of the American College of Surgeons*: "Throughout his professional life, Dr. Graham was active and very effective in training young surgeons. He was an excellent teacher; he always maintained a true academic spirit and set high professional standards for all. He expected a lot from his trainees, but treated them with the utmost respect. For these and many other reasons, they were sincerely devoted to him, as he was to them and his many, many other friends. Students from all over the world came to study under him. The great value of his inspiration and teaching is attested by the fact that many of them were selected to head surgical departments in their home countries. The same can be said about his influence on young surgeons here in America; no other American surgeon has trained so many young surgeons to be heads of departments of surgery."

As an instructor of surgery, Cole received a salary of about $1,800 a year and maintained a hospital-based private practice. Over the ten years that he spent at Washington University after his residency training, he rose through the instructor ranks to become associate professor of surgery. All the while, he continued to broaden his research projects and interests.

He even delved into such modern concerns as the effects of caffeine on the body. In a paper published in 1934, called "Effect of Caffeine on Basal Metabolism," Cole and his research colleague Nathan Womack found that caffeine increased the basal metabolism, or the basic amount of heat the body produces, of a guinea pig for almost 24 hours. Determination of basal metabolism was considered an important factor in the diagnosis of a patient thought to have hyperthyroidism, an abnormality of the thyroid gland.

Much more significant, though, were his studies, again with Dr. Womack, concerning the role of the thyroid gland in fighting disease. In a report published in the *Journal of the*

American Medical Association in 1928, the investigators concluded from a series of animal experiments: "All the data presented in this article point strongly to the fact that the thyroid gland takes an active part in the mechanisms combating diseases of the body in general. Especially does this seem true in acute infections and fevers." Here was another example of the simple observation that led to far-reaching medical consequences. Womack and Cole's other studies of the thyroid gland included a study that explored the effect of the thyroid gland on the basal metabolic rate (1928), a probe into the reaction of the thyroid gland to infections in other parts of the body (1929), and a report on normal and pathologic repair of the thyroid (1931).

"The role of the thyroid in the maintenance of body immunity against bacterial toxins and other poisons has been discussed pro and con for years," Cole and Womack wrote in the *Journal of the American Medical Association* in 1929, when little was known of the endocrine system. "Wells, McCarrison and others favor the idea that the thyroid takes an active part in the resistance of the body to many toxins. In fact, McCarrison, speaking of the thyroid, remarks that 'it exercises a protective antitoxic and immunizing action, defending the body not only against the toxic products of its own metabolism but against disease-producing microorganisms and injury by their products.' Pickworth feels that the extreme variations which he obtained in the iodine content of thyroids of patients who succumbed to acute infections indicates a very marked relation between thyroid activity and septic processes. The selective action of certain toxins and infectious processes against the thyroid (histologically and chemically) which we have observed leads us to concur strongly in these opinions."

On his own, Dr. Cole did some interesting research on appendicitis, peritonitis (a life-threatening inflammatory disease of the abdominal cavity), and bleeding in the tissue that lines the abdominal cavity.

"Appreciating the difficulty in distinguishing between retroperitoneal hemorrhage [bleeding in the abdominal cavity] and early peritonitis," Cole wrote for the *Journal of the American Medical Association* in 1931, "I sought aid from the literature but was surprised to learn that there are practically no references to retroperitoneal hemorrhage in the literature, at least during the past ten years." He made the point that abdominal bleeding sometimes masquerades as acute peritonitis caused by appendicitis.

In a related study of chronic appendicitis, which was published in 1935, Cole concluded, "The actual number of cases of chronic appendicitis is considerably smaller than generally appreciated. An enormous amount of difficulty may be experienced in arriving at a correct diagnosis because of the paucity of manifestations and the similarity of the symptoms to those caused by many other diseases. For this reason, a thorough examination of the patient is necessary. When operation is performed, the incision must be made near the midline and large enough to allow a thorough exploration of the abdominal cavity."

At about this same time, drug therapy got one of its biggest boosts with the introduction of sulfonamides, or sulfa drugs, to combat bacterial infections. The sulfa drugs were especially valuable in treating infections related to surgery, such as peritonitis, one of Cole's concerns, and empyema, Graham's big area of research. The sulfa drugs greatly lessened the incidence of empyema by attacking the bacterial causes of pneumonia. When antibiotics were discovered in the mid-1940s, empyema was almost completely eliminated and is today a rare disease. The new sulfa drugs also significantly reduced the number of deaths from appendicitis.

In another study worthy of note, Cole examined the role of a poorly functioning liver (hepatic insufficiency) in diseases that required surgery. "We are realizing more and more," he said before the annual meeting of the Missouri State Medical Association in 1933, "that hepatic insufficiency is an important symptom or complication of many diseases and that it is a very significant item from the standpoint of the surgeon in the determination of operability. Unfortunately, this condition is usually not recognizable clinically until the disease is far advanced. This insidious characteristic has led to many attempts to test for insufficiency by laboratory means and has been responsible for the development of an enormous number of laboratory tests, none of which are entirely satisfactory." He recommended that the patient's liver problems be treated before an operation is performed. "Obviously, unless operation is urgently indicated, operative procedures should be postponed until the patient has had proper restorative treatment," he said.

Along with the widespread use of the Graham-Cole test for gallbladder disease and Cole's diverse and insightful contributions to the medical literature of the time came a certain amount of fame for the young associate professor of surgery. Graham's reputation was also growing, especially after he performed his first lung removal operation. That accomplishment helped Cole as well. In the mid-1930s, a number of other medical schools began trying to woo Warren Cole away from Washington University and his chief of surgery.

"I was invited to go to Vanderbilt University in Nashville, where Barney Brooks was now teaching," Dr. Cole said in a interview after his retirement. "The offer was not for the head of the department of surgery, but they wanted me to build up the residency program there. I studied that offer for a while because it was a good one—they were grooming me for the number two position. I turned them down, though, because I was in the middle of a lot of research with Dr. Graham.

"Then I was offered a job as professor of surgery at the University of Louisville in Kentucky. The position would have led to the top spot as head of the department in a year or so. They wanted a young department head, and the person who was there wanted to resign. But I was right in the cream of my research at Washington University. Louisville was a smaller school and didn't have much money to build a department with. That was the primary reason I turned them down. I had too many roots in research in St. Louis and it was pretty hard to move on. Dr. Graham discouraged me from leaving. He always said, 'You've got a better opportunity here.'"

Then came an offer Dr. Cole could not refuse. The University of Illinois College of Medicine in Chicago wanted him as its first full-time professor of surgery. In 1934, the U. of I. had formed a special committee to fill the chair of surgery with its first full-time head of a clinical department. One Saturday night in 1935, Julius Hess, then professor of pediatrics and chairman of the special committee, called Dr. Cole in St. Louis and offered him the position.

It did not take Cole long to say yes. Even Evarts Graham blessed the move. "When the Illinois job came along, Dr. Graham said, 'Now you're ready to go,'" Cole recalled. His appointment was effective September 1, 1936.

With about 160 students in 1936, Illinois had one of the largest medical schools in the country. By 1931, with a state appropriation of $1.5 million, the university had built a new medical school complex on Chicago's west side to add to a group of hospitals and medical institutes known as the Research and Educational Hospitals, which were begun on the site in 1925. The hospitals were built by the State Department of Public Welfare and staffed by the University of Illinois. The new medical school complex also included a new psychiatric wing to the general hospital and a research laboratory and library. And the next year, even though the Great Depression was in its depths, the state came up with an additional $1.4 million for another unit of buildings in the same block to provide hospital laboratories, a college of dentistry, and facilities for the study of pathology, bacteriology and public health. In short, the University of Illinois College of Medicine had extensive teaching and research facilities to offer and strong financial backing from the state legislature.

Chicago itself was also a lure that could not be ignored. Within Warren Cole's lifetime, the city had grown to a bustling metropolis and was recognized as one of the nation's chief medical centers. It boasted three prominent medical schools—Rush Medical College, which was then affiliated with the University of Chicago, Northwestern University Medical School and the University of Illinois College of Medicine. All of the schools had embarked on large-scale building programs in the early decades of the 20th century. In fact, the facilities for medical education had grown to be so extensive in Chicago that by 1936, more third- and fourth-year medical students were being educated in Chicago than in any other U.S. city except Philadelphia.

Chicago was a center for medical organizations as well.

The American Medical Association and the American College of Surgeons, along with a number of other medical societies and associations, were headquartered in the "city of the big shoulders," as Carl Sandburg called it.

The position at the University of Illinois also offered Cole the opportunity to be the type of surgeon Evarts Graham had shown him how to be—educator, research scientist and ethical practitioner. Just how much Evarts Graham influenced Cole's life over the long term is difficult to assess accurately. Dr. Cole admittedly admired him as a role model and a great man in the field of surgery. That he chose to follow a similar path as Graham is not surprising—he was groomed for it early on by the various physicians who took part in his medical education and surgical training. But it was Graham more than any other who nurtured Cole's persona as a surgeon.

·   "We looked upon Dr. Graham as *the* knowledgeable man and tried to make ourselves like him," Dr. Cole said in his retirement years. "We watched him and copied him. Throughout residency training, we realized we had to do our jobs a little better than the other fellow to demonstrate that we were the main ones to appoint to the next position. Graham had not gone through a formal residency system and so his surgical technique was not the best. But he was smart. His strong point was research. He was able to pick up knowledge very skillfully. He read a great deal. Surgeons, as they develop, will achieve certain features of excellence by paying attention to those features that spell success in those who train them."

On August 7, 1936, Evarts Graham responded to a letter from Warren Cole in which he expressed his appreciation for all the things the chief had done for him. Graham's reply read:

"I am deeply touched by the kind things which you say, but I cannot take very much credit for your brilliant success in your splendid career. The only thing for which I perhaps might deserve some credit was the fact that I recognized a good man when I saw him, although he was at that time only a kid. I often do congratulate myself on the fact that I was able to recognize your great ability at that time.

"I feel the greatest confidence in your success at the University of Illinois and I know that we are all going to point to you with tremendous pride, but I hope that you will wish to come back once in a while. I am sure that even if you do not find an opportunity to do so, our paths will cross every once in a while at meetings. At any rate, you can feel assured that all of us here will be eagerly watching the brilliant achievements which we know you will accomplish."

And so Cole broke his ties with Washington University School of Medicine and Dr. Graham, and in September of 1936, began a new career as a full-time professor of surgery and head of the department of surgery at the University of Illinois College of Medicine in Chicago. He was 38 years old, single, and a rising young star in academic surgery. He was both excited and nervous about the opportunity that lay before him, an opportunity that allowed him to continue his research, foster the education of medical students and residents, and influence a great university and the burgeoning field of surgery.

SECTION THREE:
❧
THE UNIVERSITY OF ILLINOIS YEARS

CHAPTER 10

🙠

THE WEST SIDE STORY

W hen the redoubtable Abraham Flexner made his inspection of the 14 medical schools then in existence in Chicago in 1909, he damned the city as "the plague spot of the country" for medical education.

State law required high school education or its equivalent for entrance to medical schools, but even some of the best schools, including the University of Illinois, were interpreting the admission requirement loosely and letting in unqualified students. Flexner found that 10 of the 14 schools he visited were in flagrant violation of the law and some, he charged, with the "connivance of the state board." If higher admission standards were set, he predicted, only Rush Medical College, Northwestern University Medical School, and the College of Physicians and Surgeons—which at that time served as the medical school of the University of Illinois under a lease agreement—would survive.

Flexner found the teaching facilities at Northwestern and the College of Physicians and Surgeons "distinctly inferior" to Rush, and the clinical facilities at the College of Physicians and Surgeons somewhat inferior to Northwestern and Rush, although all three schools used the city's public hospital, Cook County Hospital, for their clinical instruction. However, Flexner saved his sharpest criticism for the ten substandard day and evening schools that he found operating in Chicago. Most of these schools were diploma mills that accepted any amount of education as equivalent to a high school degree, and none of them offered anything like adequate clinical training. In fact, several of the evening schools offered courses in anatomy without providing dissection facilities.

The effect of Flexner's report was shattering to most of the medical schools in Chicago. The better schools moved quickly to raise admission standards and improve their teaching facilities. Within 15 years after Flexner's report was published, the medical schools that survived made tremendous strides in bringing their levels of education up to the best criteria of contemporary medical instruction. Schools began requiring two years of college and then three years for admission to medical training, and they began to insist on a high level of scholastic achievement from their incoming students.

Before 1918, none of the schools required a compulsory internship, but in that year Rush Medical College offered its senior students a choice of an internship or a fifth year of advanced study in a clinical department. In 1922, the Illinois State Medical Society required every graduating medical student to serve a one-year internship in a hospital of at least 25 beds.

The Flexner report also prodded medical schools into affiliations with universities. So in 1913, the College of Physicians and Surgeons, which up until that point had been a proprietary school owned by its faculty, was joined permanently to the University of Illinois and became known as the University of Illinois College of Medicine.

The original College of Physicians and Surgeons was formed in 1881 by a group of five physicians who incorporated the school as a proprietary venture, issued $30,000 in stock and bought up all the initial stock themselves. They then sold faculty positions and part ownership in the institution for the price of $2,000 for a professorship and $500 for a lectureship. The school had to be run on the fees collected from students, and the faculty received most of their income from private practice. The only admission requirements were that applicants had to be 18 years old and of good moral character and had to pass some sort of entrance exam. Although the curriculum was three years long, attendance was required at only two annual courses of lectures that each lasted six months.

The founders financed a four-story Queen Anne style building for the new college to be built across the street from Cook County Hospital, which had been relocated to the west side of the city after the Great Fire of 1871 ravaged its former building along the lakefront to the east. The new college building included the West Side Free Dispensary, which was an early version of an outpatient clinic; a huge lecture room that seated 226; a large operating room; a library; and laboratories for chemistry and physiology.

In 1891, surgeon Bayard Holmes came on the faculty as education director, beefed up the laboratory classes in the basic sciences curriculum and persuaded the powers that were to build a six-story lab building adjacent to the main structure. The school's lab courses began to rival those offered at the University of Michigan and Eastern medical schools, and its bacteriology course was the first one ever offered in a Chicago medical school.

This new emphasis on lab teaching put the College of Physicians and Surgeons in the vanguard of medical education and attracted more and more students. After the turn of the century, the school added what it called elementary clinics to the basic science curriculum in an effort to introduce the first- and second-year students to clinical medicine.

Efforts had been made in the 1890s by the governor of the state to have the University of Illinois acquire the College of Physicians and Surgeons, but the state legislature voted down the appropriations bill. As an alternative, the board of trustees of the university approved a contract to lease the College of Physicians and Surgeons for its department of medicine. Financially, the arrangement was a good deal for the university, and the contract remained in effect until 1912 when the College went off on its own again. But in 1913, recognizing a need to be connected to a university, the faculty and alumni of the College of Physicians and Surgeons bought up all the stock of the school and presented it gratis to the board of trustees of the University of Illinois.

The trustees immediately came up with $100,000 to strengthen the basic science courses, and the university began to hire full-time faculty for the preclinical years. Entrance requirements were raised at first to 30 hours of college credit and then to 60, and incoming students had to have taken two years of chemistry and two years of French or German, as well as one year each of biology and physics. As a result, enrollment plummeted, from 158 in 1912 to 13 in 1914. The College of Medicine recovered, along with the other schools that raised entrance requirements in the post-Flexner era, when the nation's high school system caught up to medical school requirements. Educators in general rejoiced in the transition.

By 1919, the College's building across the street from Cook County Hospital was so cramped and outmoded that the College of Medicine struck a deal with the State Department of Public Welfare to the effect that Public Welfare would build and maintain a group of research and education hospitals and the College would staff them. So the state bought up a big-league baseball field in the same neighborhood, where the Chicago Cubs had played from 1893 until 1916. It became the center of the new University of Illinois College of Medicine.

By the time Dr. Cole arrived in 1936, most of the buildings of the medical center were completed and the medical school was just beginning to build up its clinical faculty. On the occasion of the 100th anniversary of the medical school in 1981, Dr. Joseph Kiefer, a urology professor, recalled what the medical center was like in the 1930s:

"Like a medieval university in a European town, the medical center was an enclave set down in the center of what was essentially a southern Italian or Sicilian village. The neighborhood was filled with older two- and three-flat apartment buildings in varying states of repair or disrepair, owned and occupied mostly by middle and lower income Italians who worked hard to pay off their mortgages or to start small businesses and stores, often restaurants, which were the most common meeting places of the two cultures.

"The area was also a recruiting ground for organized crime; one might find them eating at adjoining tables at the local restaurants. The attitude of the local inhabitants toward the medical people was not hostility but rather respect, which sometimes extended itself to protectiveness. Nurses or house staff in 'whites' or others identified by a medical or OB bag could walk the streets of the area without fear. Mugging or strong-arming of medical personnel was unheard of."

Writing in 1981 for the same centennial issue of the *Scope*, the alumni magazine of the medical school, Dr. Cole remembered what conditions were like when he arrived at the ballpark-turned-medical-center on the west side of Chicago: "From the Washington University Medical School, I came to the University of Illinois as head of the department of surgery on September 1, 1936. I was the first full-time head of a clinical department at the U. of I. Since only a minority of the heads of the clinical departments in state medical schools were full time then, it might be said that this assignment was a bit experimental. I was the only full-time member of the department.

"When I came to Illinois I was quite disappointed in the space assigned to the department. Besides a room for myself and a secretary, we had only one or two small rooms for staff members. The DMP [Dentistry, Medicine, Pharmacy] building appeared quite large, but it was apparently customary for the clinical departments to be housed in the hospital, which was at that time quite small (about 225 beds). This number of beds was really much too small for the large class of students (about 160; the school was among the largest in the country). We could use Cook County Hospital but only for patients for lectures and not clinical clerkships. As a consequence, we clinicians began talking about an addition to the hospital, but such was not obtained until 1953. This lack of patients for our large class encouraged me to request other hospitals, including Presbyterian, St. Luke's, Illinois Central and one or two others, to help with the surgical teaching.

"At the time of my arrival at the U. of I., much of the teaching in all medical schools was of the didactic type, even though clerkships on the wards had been introduced many years previously. Illinois was no exception to the didactic custom. Three or four members of the surgical staff, including the late Drs. Phifer, Post and Bamberger, conducted a didactic course which was very strict, with several failures each quarter (but apparently not as bad as Michigan, where, rumor had it, 20 to 25 percent of the junior class failed). The students were displeased with this course, but after graduation many told me they were glad it was so tough because they 'sure learned a lot of surgery.'"

The idea of a full-time clinical faculty was a hotly debated one even when Cole was appointed to his post in 1936. In the years after Flexner, much of the funding for medical schools went to research, and those funds allowed the creation of new positions in academic medicine. Rockefeller's philanthropic arm, the General Education Board, was the greatest proponent of the strict full-time system as implemented at Johns Hopkins, and its moneys flowed to schools that followed the plan. The strict full-time plan meant that the faculty member's salary came solely from teaching and research without outside consulting. Harvard University and many other schools advocated instead the geographic full-time system in which professors were allowed to retain consulting fees as a economic incentive for carrying on their work but saw private patients only in their university hospitals.

One of the harshest critics of the salaried full-time plan was Arthur Dean Bevan. Bevan was professor of surgery at Rush Medical College in Chicago and enormously powerful as chairman of the Council on Medical Education of the American Medical Association, which was one of the prime forces behind reform in medical education in this country. Bevan felt that the General Education Board had become a "disturbing influence by dictating the scheme of organization of our medical schools." But despite the controversy over the two forms of full time and despite the length of time it took to implement the full-time system in clinical medical education, most physicians in academia believed that the system was worthwhile. The principle behind the system was that the clinical professor's role was to concentrate on teaching and research and not on building up a practice.

Dr. Cole was hired at the University of Illinois on a strict full time basis, even though geographic full time was the scheme in force in most medical schools at the time. He received a salary only and was not allowed to earn income from treating patients. Teaching and research became the center of his academic life.

In a speech given in 1941, when he was made president of the prestigious Society of University Surgeons, Warren Cole talked about the importance of research in the life of an academic surgeon. Cole quoted from physiologist Claude Bernard, who, in 1865, wrote a book called *Experimental Medicine*, which Cole called a masterpiece on the philosophy of research: "Experimentation is undeniably harder in medicine than in any other science; but for that very reason it was never so necessary, and indeed so indispensable. The more complex the science, the more essential it is, in fact, to establish a good experimental standard, so as to secure comparable facts, free from sources of error. Nothing, I believe, is today so important to the progress of medicine."

In the same 1941 speech, Cole expressed his own ideas about the value of constant research to expand the borders of medicine. "The young ambitious medical scientist, more saturated perhaps with the vision of glory than with the persevering, analytic astuteness of a seasoned scientist, may in desperation and disgust say, 'Why work anymore; all discoveries of importance have already been made?' Of course, we are all aware of the fallacy of that remark and realize that the addition of scientific facts as compiled year after year increases the chances of development of epoch-making discoveries in geometric ratio. True enough, the chances of making epochal discoveries in the mechanics of operative principles are being diminished; not so, though, with the physiologic principles which can be utilized for the patient's welfare before or after operative procedures are performed.

"As all of us fully realize, the benefits derived from the practice of medicine or surgery may be threefold: personal satisfaction or happiness, financial reward, and creation of an enviable professional reputation. All of the peers and seers of medicine as far back as the Hippocratic era remind us of the serious accusations hurled at the monetary instinct. It is axiomatic that indeed few surgeons of the academic group (exemplified by this society) chose that path for the monetary compensation obtainable. Naturally, they elected to spend the majority of their time in institutional work for the personal satisfaction derived from the work itself or the reputation created. I have no doubt that all the members of this audience are well aware of the curious fact that the shortcut to an enviable national reputation lies in the corridors which traverse the halls of experimental medicine and surgery. The esteem of one's fellows, beyond his local environs, can be achieved in about half the time required by concentration on purely clinical medicine or surgery. It is likewise self-evident that because of his lasting contributions to mankind, this type of doctor will always be in demand. May his kind flourish and prosper!"

Cole fell heir to a long line of talented surgeons who had occupied the chair of surgery at one time or another in the 55-year history of the medical school affiliated with the University of Illinois. Among the most famous was John B. Murphy, a Wisconsin farm boy who grew up to be what many surgeons considered the finest teacher and operator of his day. He drew national fame when he treated Teddy Roosevelt for a gunshot wound the former President suffered in Milwaukee in 1912. Murphy was a sort of man for all seasons in surgery; there was virtually no field of surgery to which he did not make some significant contribution. In 1892, he devised the Murphy button, which was a metal button about the size of a doughnut hole that helped surgeons suture together two cut-open ends of the intestine. He railed against fee-splitting and was almost impeached while president of the Chicago Medical Society. Many admired him and many more envied him.

Cole's immediate predecessor as head of surgery at Illinois was Dr. Carl A. Hedblom, who died at age 55 in 1934. Hedblom had gotten his MD degree from Harvard in 1911 and a PhD from the Mayo Foundation at the University of Minnesota in 1920. He served as professor of surgery at the Harvard Medical School in China from 1913 to 1916, and was a staff surgeon at the Mayo Clinic from 1918 to 1924. Prior to becoming head of the department of surgery at the University of Illinois in 1926, Hedblom had held the same position at the University of Wisconsin for two years. While at Illinois, he was also surgeon-in-chief at the university's Research and Educational Hospitals. Hedblom was a strong clinical surgeon who focused on teaching and patient care.

But the full-time chief of surgery appointed in 1936 was a new breed, a clinical scientist through and through who delighted and found his rewards in the lab, not in the limelight of surgical practice. He had a different philosophy and orientation than his predecessors. His goal was teaching and research and his style was meticulous and methodical, not flamboyant and flashy. Cole's domain was in "the halls of experimental research and surgery" while others found fame in the corridors filled with operating rooms. In 1936, he set out to build a program of clinical surgery at the University of Illinois in the rich tradition of the medical schools at Johns Hopkins and Washington University. He spent the next 30 years of his life doing just that, along the way gaining an enviable national and international reputation.

Throughout the late 1930s and early 1940s, the medical center at the University of Illinois grew in size and stature. An addition to the medical and dental college laboratory building went up in 1937, and by 1940 the Department of Welfare had completed an annex to the Institute for Crippled Children and a new Neuropsychiatric Institute as part of the Research and Educational Hospitals. In 1941, the Illinois state legislature authorized the creation of a special medical center district with power to buy land and clear slums on the west side of Chicago.

The nucleus of the district was the University of Illinois, with its hospitals, institutes, and schools of medicine, dentistry and pharmacy, along with Cook County Hospital, Presbyterian Hospital, and two other medical schools—Loyola University School of Medicine and the Chicago Medical School. New projects planned for the district were a Veterans Administration hospital, a new campus for Loyola's medical and dental schools, a state-run tuberculosis hospital and research institute, and a graduate school of medicine run by Cook County. In 1941, Rush Medical College, Chicago's oldest medical school, ended its affiliation with the University of Chicago and its faculty members joined the University of Illinois medical faculty.

To this buzz of activity and expansive growth, Warren Cole added his own research beehive in surgery. When his predecessor, Dr. Carl Hedblom, gave his last annual report to the dean of the College of Medicine in 1934, he devoted it to a discussion of the progress made in the diagnosis and treatment of disease and the need for surgeons to specialize in a specific aspect of surgery because of the tremendous growth of knowledge in the field.

"Intensive studies of the outward manifestations of morbid processes and of the changes produced by them as found not only post mortem but also in the living at operation and animal experimentation has added so enormously to our knowledge of their nature, prevention and treatment that it is no longer possible for any one surgeon to keep abreast of progress, to master all the difficult diagnostic procedures...to become skilled in the practical application of all the technical operative procedures," Dr. Hedblom wrote in his annual report. "Only by limiting himself to a special field is the surgeon able to give to the patient the best that modern surgery has to offer and only so is he able to make any important contributions to it. Leaders and masters in surgery of necessity have become specialists." Hedblom then described the activities of the various branches of the department of surgery— neurological, oral, thoracic, genitourinary, orthopaedic and general surgery—with reference to teaching and clinical and experimental research.

Dr. Cole's annual report to Dean David J. Davis in 1941, on the other hand, spoke only of experimental research. He specifically listed 21 research projects in progress, studies that touched an amazing variety of surgical topics, including how various drugs affect the movement of the intestine, the effect of shock on liver function, what causes negative reactions from blood transfusions, the beneficial effects of vitamin K on jaundice, the effect of amino acids on protein metabolism, the action of a sulfa drug on bacteria in the intestine, and the relationship between vitamin B-1 deficiencies and deaths from surgery.

Cole himself was involved with residents and staff in studies of the use of cortin (an adrenal gland extract) in the prevention and treatment of shock, the effects of vitamin C and a sulfa drug on disease and death from surgery, a new operation for anal stricture in infants, and a metabolic study involving a new method that Cole devised of concocting a cholesterol emulsion for intravenous injections.

In addition, he published the third edition of his *Textbook of General Surgery*, which he co-authored with Dr. Robert Elman, professor of clinical surgery at Washington University School of Medicine. The first edition was published in 1936, the year he went to Illinois, and was dedicated to Evarts Graham, "teacher, chief and friend, who has exerted a guiding influence for many years on our professional careers."

In the same year, Cole also published articles on the pancreatic hepatic syndrome, precautions in thyroid surgery, laboratory aids in surgery, prerequisites in thyroid surgery, and current concepts in handling gallbladder disease, along with several book reviews. Warren Cole as educator, researcher and medical leader was in his stride.

Chapter 11

?&

The Woman Who Came Down the Hall

W hatever plans Dr. Cole, the University of Illinois and the rest of the country, for that matter, had for the future in the early 1940s were inexorably changed on December 7, 1941, when the Japanese bombed Pearl Harbor and the United States entered World War II.

On January 28, 1942, shortly after the attack, Dr. Cole was asked to describe the medical lessons learned from the assault before a meeting of the faculty at the U. of I. medical center. "An important feature in the attack upon Pearl Harbor," Cole said, "was that about half of the casualties were burns. Burns are very painful, and this number emphasized the advantage of syrettes of morphine instead of tablets for hypodermic use. Sulfanilamide [a sulfa drug] was used freely in all wounds as soon as aid could reach the wounded soldier. Several grams were dumped into the wounds and sterile dressings applied. Since abdominal and brain injuries received first care in the hospitals, many soft-tissue wounds, as well as compound fractures, had to be delayed 12 to 48 hours for operative therapy. It was found that compound fractures could be debrided as long as 48 hours after injury if sulfanilamide had been placed in the wound and had been given regularly up to the time of operation. They were also treated by the oral method utilizing debridement, reduction, packing with vaseline gauze and sulfanilamide, followed immediately by plaster cast. No significant infections occurred in any of the compound fractures treated in this way. Small soft-tissue wounds were closed, but large wounds were packed open. Infections in such wounds were trivial; many were closed by secondary suture after several days."

In his 1942 annual report to the president of the University of Illinois, the dean of the College of Medicine, David Davis, described how the medical school was affected by the war. "Throughout the year the work in the College has been dominated by special war activities. For example, changes from the semester to the quarter schedule have been initiated. Beginning in June 1942, the accelerated program will be inaugurated with the junior and senior students returning for summer work. It is the plan of the College to cooperate with the war program in every way possible. The students have been requested to apply for commissions in the Army or Navy Medical Corps Reserve and all have done so.

"To date, over 70 of our faculty members have been called for active military duty. We anticipate that many more of our younger men will be called soon. A hospital unit is being formed at this time, with Lt. Col. Charles B. Puestow, M.D., Associate Professor of Surgery, in charge. It is expected that about 40 additional members of our staff will be included in this group.

"The College was called upon to submit to the Procurement and Assignment Service, Washington, D.C., a complete list in which all faculty and staff members were classified as either 'essential' or 'available.' So far our essential classifications have been respected and given full consideration by the various war agencies. However, at the present time a reclassification, especially for those members under 45 years of age, is being made with a view to decreasing more and more the number of people considered 'essential' to the teaching program and the maintenance of the dispensary and hospital work."

Dr. Cole was one of the faculty members considered essential but he nonetheless wanted to go to war. "Many heads of departments of surgery throughout the United States organized a military unit (usually in the Army) named after the universities to which they were attached, and went into military service," Cole wrote in his retirement years. "Very soon after World War II started, I wrote to General Rankin, who was assigned by the Surgeon General to help with placement of medical personnel, asking what he wanted me to do. Instead of suggesting I head up some sort of military unit, he told me by mail he rather decisively wanted me to stay in Chicago, and with the small unit of personnel we had left in Chicago, wanted me to turn out as many graduate M.D.'s as we could every nine months."

Brigadier General Fred W. Rankin's letter to Warren Cole, dated March 19, 1942, read in part: "I really feel that you are essential in the production of young medical men at the University of Illinois. We must turn out the present day maximum of physicians, and we must do this without lowering of standards. You have a growing institution which has made great strides and I am sure that your part in this progress has been a large one."

A year later, Cole tried once again to get into the Army. Once again, General Rankin turned him down, in a letter dated March 11, 1943: "I know you want to get into the Army. It is a perfectly natural and patriotic desire, but everybody can't wear a uniform and it looks as though your particular job is to continue teaching. If the war lasts long enough maybe you will get your chance, but right now be satisfied where you are."

But while he was itching to go to war, Dr. Cole established a new beachhead on the home front. Despite his shyness with women and his long bachelorhood, Warren Cole, at age 43, married Mrs. Clara M. Lund, 38, a widow, on June 13, 1942. The two had met by chance in a large apartment building on Chicago's lakefront, where they both lived. Dr. Cole described the meeting and courtship in an essay entitled "How to Choose a Bride with Happy Results" written when he was in his retirement years.

"I have a batting average of one hundred percent in this enterprise, but you might question the importance of this figure by inquiring about the length of my series. Yes, you are right—-the series is only one.

"I gave no thought to getting married while I was in

medical school, and not even while I was in residency training. Dr. Graham had no rule against marriage while I was in surgical training, but all residents knew he frowned upon the idea. Having some effect on the idea was the belief of Dr. Barney Brooks on Dr. Graham's staff that if he were head of a department and a resident got married, he would fire the resident. During my time working in the department of surgery, I had met several girls (mostly nurses) whom I continued to see off and on, but none of these appeared to be the one I wanted to marry.

"Dr. Graham and I were so busy with problems related to cholecystography for several years after we opened this box that I really had no time to think about getting married. As a matter of fact, I gave no serious thought to the problem until I accepted the headship of the department of surgery at the University of Illinois in 1936, at the age of 38. By that time I had no objections to the idea, but it seems I had never met the right girl. But I continued to be neutral to the idea.

"When I moved to Chicago, I naturally looked around for and inquired of friends about living quarters. I chose a huge apartment house at 1400 Lake Shore Drive. One day when I was coming home from work and walking down the hall toward the elevators, I got the shock of my life. Walking towards me was a young woman. I glanced at her to see if I knew her. She was a good-looking young woman, perhaps in her early thirties. I stopped in my tracks. I glanced at her a second time. Yes, there could be no question about it—she was the girl I was going to marry or at least would want to marry.

"It was amazing to me that I should get such an idea after merely meeting her in the hall. After we passed in the hall, I stepped over to the newspaper stand of the gift shop and asked who that lady was. Yes, the man at the stand knew her. Her name was Lund, her husband had died a couple of years ago, and she worked at the *Chicago Daily News*. I stopped for mail and then went up to my apartment. That face was stamped indelibly in my mind. I could not erase it. I went down to the dining room about 6:30 pm. I was led to a table by the head waitress and I sat down. Yes, then I looked around to see if she was there. No, she was not. I glanced through my newspaper, not remembering what I had read. I ate my dinner with my usual lack of appetite (or less) and retired to my apartment. I went over the homework I had brought from my office. Yes, I found it very uninteresting.

"I slept poorly that night; the face of the woman I had met in the hall kept flashing through my mind. The next evening I hurried into the hall of my apartment building, hoping I would see that attractive face once more. A few days later I met her again. Yes, there was no doubt about it, she was the one I wanted to marry. After seeing her a few times after that, I asked the man at the newspaper stand if he would introduce me to the young lady he told me was employed by the *Chicago Daily News*. This he did a few evenings later.

"She exhibited very little interest in our introduction. Strange to say, this bothered me very little because I was not looking for a woman who would be thrilled with meeting every eligible bachelor she could find. I asked if I might call her. She did not reply to this. Nevertheless, I called her a few days later and really had to talk her into going out with me for dinner. I now discovered I had fallen in love with the lady. She told me she was not thrilled with meeting young men. I could understand that a good-looking young lady like her would get calls from innumerable young men—so many calls that she was not interested in them.

"After we spent a few more evenings together, I noted that she was interested in me, and in fact sometime later noted that she was in love with me. Shortly after that we got married. I have always been glad that I married her. She has been a wonderful wife, fulfilling all the hopes and expectations I might have for a wife.

"Very soon after our marriage, I noted she was trying to adapt to being a physician's wife, which is necessary for any woman in a marriage to a physician because that life is different. If that difference is not recognized, the marriage is apt to be ruined. Physicians in an academic life such as mine was must work extra time at night to compete successfully with associates. Physicians in practice must be subject to emergency calls. Clara understood the necessity of my working so many evenings in the week. Fortunately, she has been willing to travel with me on trips to meetings. Thus we did not have to do a lot of traveling in our later life, which often results in unfortunate complications.

"We have had no children. Shortly after our marriage, Clara had to have a hysterectomy. Knowing that this operation was essential, we did not let the lack of children interfere with our happiness. Clara is a fine cook, never complaining about that obligation. I have tried to help a bit with household necessities. We have had very few arguments. Our happiness seems to become more deeply established as the years go by. Yes, we have had a happy marriage, mostly due to her willingness to be a physician's wife. How lucky I have been, and so grateful for recognizing that she was the woman for me when I first met her in the hall 43 years ago."

A 1956 story about Dr. Cole in the *Illinois Alumni News*, a publication of the University of Illinois, has it that Cole dictated manuscripts up until 3:30 in the afternoon on the day of his own wedding at 4:00 and then left his office commenting that "I'll have to hurry because I must stop and get the ring." In an interview in 1989, Clara Cole recalled fondly that the newlyweds spent their honeymoon trout fishing. "We drove up to Land O'Lakes, Wisconsin, then across the border to the Ontonagon River in Michigan, just below the falls. Warren had a skillet in the back of the car, so he cooked my lunch when he caught the first trout. He gave me a fly rod, but he didn't give me anything to put my fish in. Then after he gave me instructions on how to cast for about half an hour, he went around a bend in the river and left me all alone. When he came back, he was surprised to find I had caught a 10-inch trout."

"To do that the first time you fish," Dr. Cole interrupted, "that's not luck, that's talent."

"We had an old Indian guide," Mrs. Cole continued, "and every year on the day after commencement, we would go to the same place to fish. It was very romantic."

But while domestic tranquility ruled the Cole household, the world around was still plunged in war. In the summer of 1941, President Franklin Roosevelt, anticipating American involvement in the war in Europe, ordered the creation of the Office of Scientific Research and Development under the National Research Council to bring the best scientific minds together to deal with the problems of war and national defense. Dr. Cole was never called to active duty, but in 1942 he was appointed secretary of the Committee on Surgery, which was set up by the Surgeon General of the United States as a unit of the Office of Scientific Research and Development's Committee on Medical Research. The purpose of the Committee on Surgery was to set standards of surgical care for victims of war and to act as an advisory group to the Surgeon General on controversial medical treatments related to surgery.

Cole's old boss, Evarts Graham, was chairman of the committee and his old college chum, Alton Ochsner, was one of about 20 top-ranking surgeons who were members. Some of the other members were Donald Balfour, professor of surgery at the University of Minnesota; Frederick Coller, professor of surgery at the University of Michigan; Howard Naffziger, professor of surgery at the University of California, San Francisco; I.S. Ravdin, professor of surgery at the University of Pennsylvania; and Allen Whipple, professor of surgery at Columbia University in New York.

"One of the most important undecided problems at the time," Dr. Cole said of his experience with the committee, "was how antibiotics should be used. Should certain amounts of a drug like sulfadiazine be sprinkled in the wound at the end of a debridement operation [the cutting away of dead tissue] or should chemotherapy be given systemically instead? At that time, Dr. Frank Meleney of Columbia University in New York was working on chemotherapy and was probably the most distinguished surgeon working in the field. Our committee asked Dr. Meleney to conduct some animal experiments comparing the results of local versus systemic treatment.

"After a year or more of studying the results obtained by various surgeons working in this field, our committee concluded that local treatment was inferior to the systemic method, although there were certain occasions when it might be superior (for example, for massive contamination). Likewise, largely because Dr. Meleney was opposed to prophylactic therapy following minor contamination, our committee did not recommend the universal use of prophylactic chemotherapy for minor bacterial contamination."

The minutes of a one of the committee's meetings, recorded by Dr. Cole, give an insight into how the group gathered and assessed information on one of the most important medical topics of the day—wound infection. The meeting took place on October 23, 1943, at the headquarters of the National Research Council in Washington, D.C.

"The Chairman introduced Major General Ogilvie, Chief Surgical Consultant of the British Eighth Army, who had recently arrived in this country. He stated that all agreed as to the life-saving qualities of sulfonamides, although he had no definite answer on the local use of the drug. They did not ask the soldier to apply or take the drug himself. However, the medical service has tried to make sulfonamide therapy universal. Their usual method is to apply it locally after debridement. He was of the opinion that the meticulous excision of the wound as developed in the last war was not necessary or indicated, since the procedure would prolong the operation and increase the tendency towards shock and tissue damage. There is a definite improvement in immobilization, transportation, health, etc., in this war. They limit the use of local sulfonamide to a maximum dose of 10 grams. By leaving the wounds open, the serious infections encountered in the last war are largely eliminated. As a rule, they give the sulfonamide by mouth for five days after infliction of the wound. Sulfanilamide is the drug of choice, since they have little sulfadiazine."

General Ogilvie was referring to the major lesson learned by surgeons in World War I: It is better to debride a contaminated wound and delay closing the wound than to close the wound immediately after debridement. Debridement and open wound management became standard practice during the first world war because many lives were saved. But it wasn't until World War II that drug therapy was available to combat wound infections. The second world war was the first war in which deaths from military action actually outnumbered deaths from disease, largely because of the availability of drugs to treat infections after the wounded tissue was debrided.

In a speech before the Mississippi Valley Medical Society in 1944, Dr. Cole explained the differences between the treatment of wounds resulting from combat versus wounds suffered in civilian life. "The treatment of wounds represents a field of surgery in which there is marked difference between civilian and military surgery," he said. "The major difference lies in the fact that in civilian surgery, practically all wounds sustained within eight to ten hours previous to treatment are closed tightly after debridement. In war, no wounds dare be closed except superficial ones which have been very recently inflicted and in which there is no contamination. Such circumstances are never encountered in wounds inflicted by exploding shells. The danger of closure of military wounds lies in the high incidence of development of severe infection, including gas gangrene. This factor was being appreciated at the close of World War I, but thousands of men undoubtedly lost their lives before this fact was understood. The importance of this feature was sharply emphasized by the fact that of 11 cases of gas gangrene encountered following the Pearl Harbor attack, all occurred in wounds which had been closed. There are obvious exceptions in military surgery, inasmuch as wounds of the peritoneal cavity, thoracic cavity and brain must be closed.

"Debridement remains as one of the most important factors in the treatment of wounds in military life as well as civilian life," Dr. Cole continued. "Proper debridement is probably even more important in war wounds, since the amount of contamination and destruction of tissues is much greater than in civilian wounds. It has been noted, time after time in this war, particularly in the North African campaign, that failure to do proper debridement resulted in a high incidence of infections."

Sulfanilamide was discovered in the mid-1930s, and numerous derivatives—the sulfa drugs—were quickly synthesized and tested for their effectiveness against various microorganisms. Studies showed that the sulfa drugs did not actually kill bacteria directly, but they arrested the growth of bacteria and allowed the body's natural defenses to finish the job. Cole's Committee on Surgery evaluated the best method of administering sulfa drugs, whether to apply them directly to the area surrounding the wound or to give them to the patient orally so that they got into the bloodstream. The committee found that oral administration was the better approach in most cases. This conclusion remained valid when penicillin and related antibiotics were put to use to fight infection toward the end of World War II.

Very little else in the history of 20th century medicine has had as great an impact on medical and surgical care as the introduction of penicillin. Alexander Fleming is credited with discovering, in London in 1928, that a lowly mold produces a substance that inhibits the growth of organisms that cause some common infectious diseases, a substance he called penicillin. Fleming's research was almost forgotten, however, until World War II when a group of Oxford scientists brought the drug to the attention of the National Research Council in Washington to obtain money and equipment for further research. The mass production of penicillin took a gargantuan cooperative effort from specialists in biology and agriculture and by government laboratories and pharmaceutical companies, all under the aegis of the Committee on Medical Research of the Office of Scientific Research and Development, which included Cole's Committee on Surgery. Unfortunately, it took until nearly the end of the war before massive quantities of penicillin were available to treat wound infections. However, the drug and its relatives soon replaced sulfa drugs because penicillin was more effective and better tolerated by the injured patient.

In the history of mankind, infections and infectious diseases have been among the major scourges of life. The work accomplished by the Committee on Medical Research and its Committee on Surgery and other subcommittees during World War II has had far-reaching implications for the treatment of a broad range of infections, including the staphylococcal infections related to surgery. The advent of sulfa drugs and the commercial development of penicillin mark the beginning of an all-out war against wound infection that, so far at least, medical science seems to be winning.

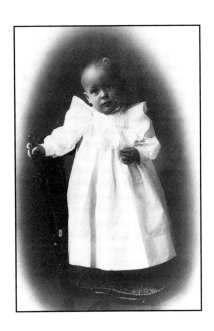

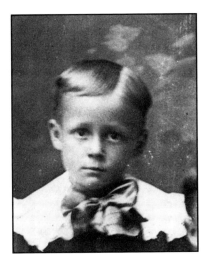

Among the earliest photos of Warren Cole are these taken when he was an infant and in his preschool days just after the turn of the century.

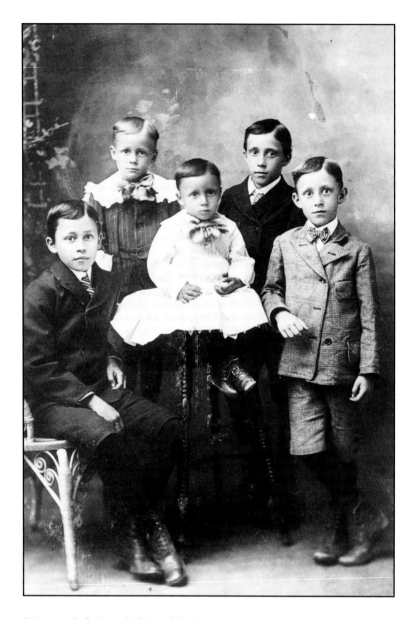

Warren Cole (top left) and his brothers: Cecil (top right), Louis (center), Perry (bottom left) and Irvin (bottom right).

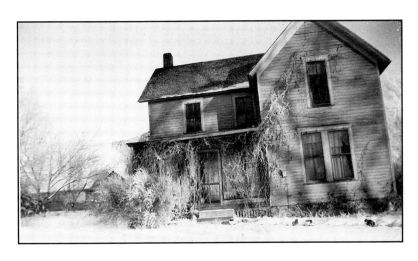

The front and east side of the Cole family farmhouse in Clay Center, Kansas.

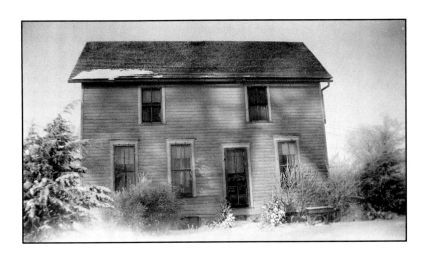

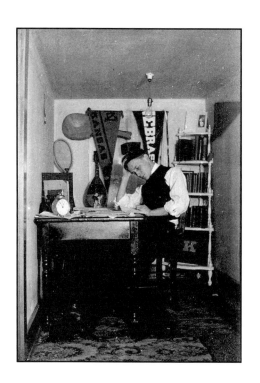

Warren Cole in 1914, studying in a corner of his room on Mississippi Avenue in Lawrence, Kansas, while he was a student at the University of Kansas. Bottom photo (undated) shows his University of Kansas yearbook picture.

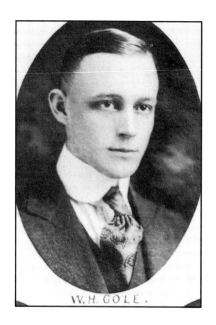

W. H. COLE.

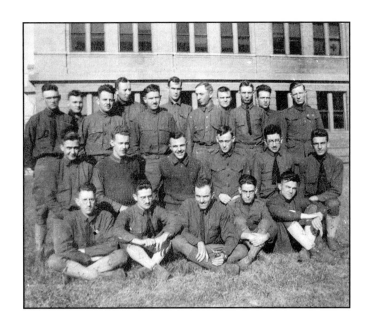

Warren in his senior year of medical school in 1919 while in the Army Reserve (third from right in the middle row) and as an intern at Baltimore City Hospitals in 1921 (back row, extreme left). Dr. Thomas Boggs is second from right in the front row.

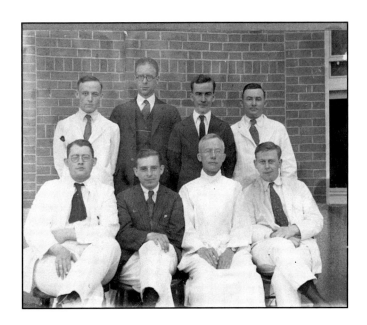

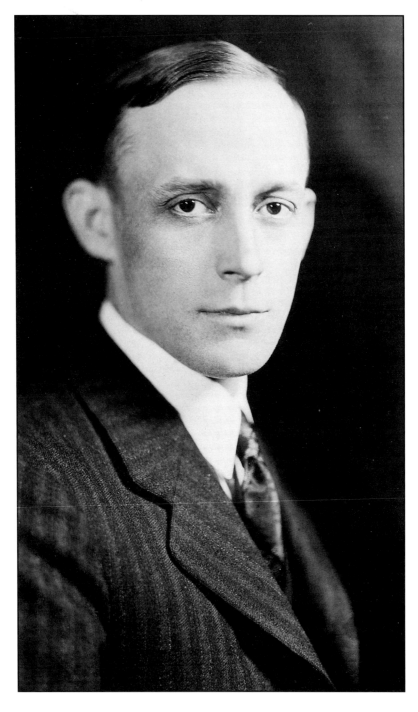

The young Dr. Warren Cole at Washington University School of Medicine in St. Louis. Undated photograph believed taken in the late 1920s or early 1930s.

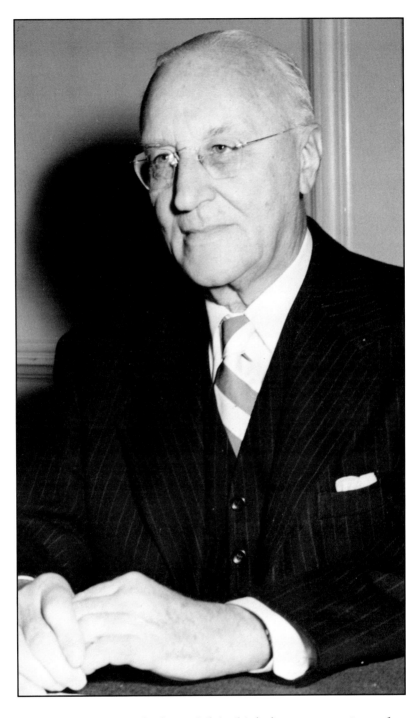

The great Dr. Evarts Graham, Cole's chief of surgery, mentor and role model. Undated photograph believed taken in the early 1950s.

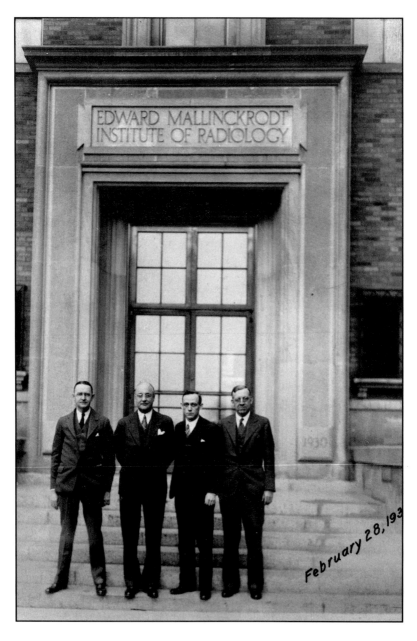

Warren Cole (right center) standing with Evarts Graham (left center) in front of the Mallinckrodt Institute of Radiology at Washington University School of Medicine in 1935. (Courtesy of the University Library Archives, University of Illinois at Chicago.)

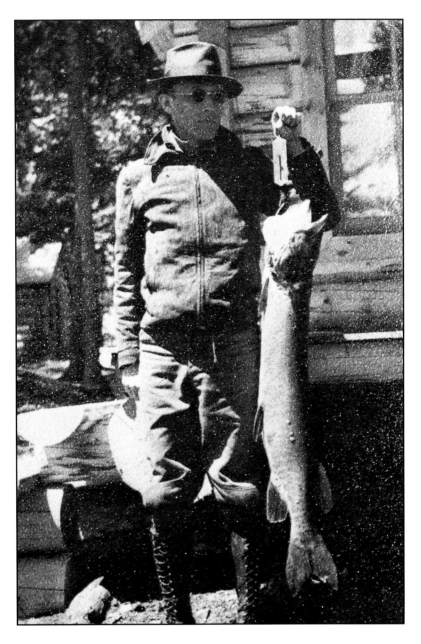

Cole at his favorite pastime with the one that didn't get away.
Undated photograph.

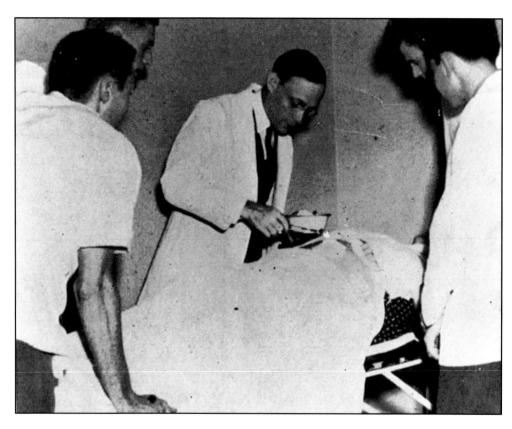

Dr. Cole attending a patient while on rounds with medical students from the University of Illinois College of Medicine in 1947. (From Illio yearbook, courtesy of the University Library Archives, University of Illinois at Chicago.)

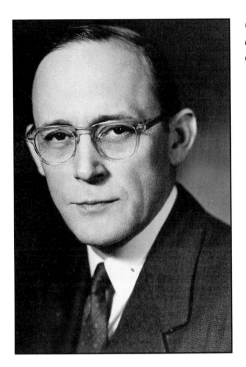

Cole in 1954 when he was doing important work in cancer.

Cole's lifelong friend, Alton Ochsner, a founder of the Ochsner Medical Institutions in New Orleans. Undated photo believed taken in the 1950s, courtesy of the American College of Surgeons archives.

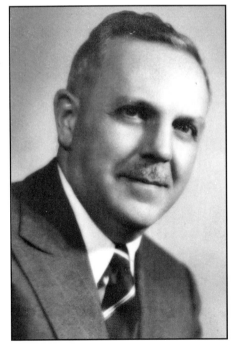

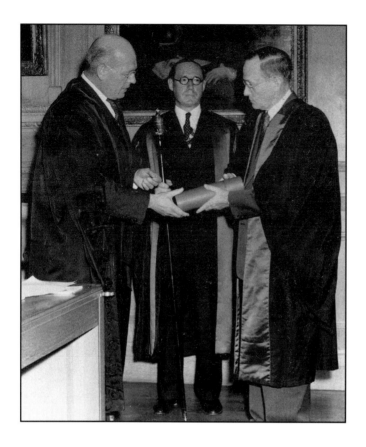

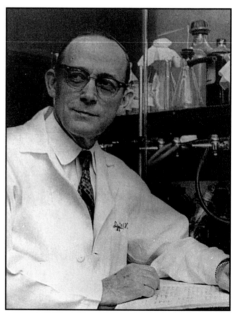

Cole receiving honorary fellowship from Sir James Paterson Ross, president of the Royal College of Surgeons of England, on July 10, 1958. At right is Cole in his lab at the University of Illinois in an undated photo believed taken in the early 1960s.

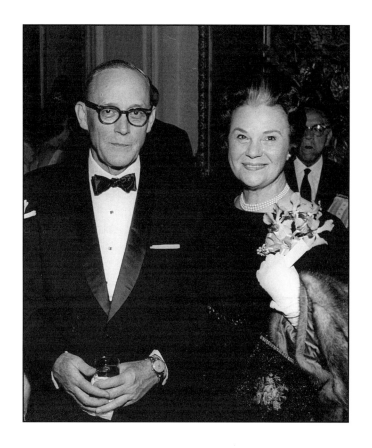

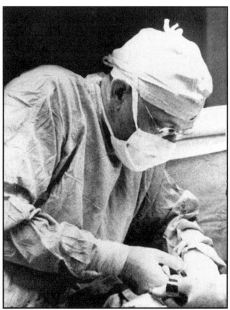

Warren and Clara Cole in 1966, the year he retired from the University of Illinois. At left is Cole in surgery in 1960. (Courtesy of the University Library Archives, University of Illinois at Chicago.)

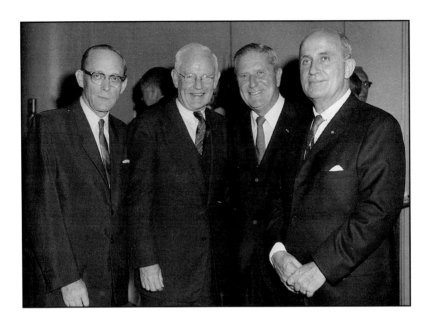

Top photo shows Dr. Cole in 1962 (left) with three former presidents of the American College of Surgeons (from left): J. Englebert Dunphy, Loyal Davis, and Robert M. Zollinger, who collaborated with Cole on a textbook of surgery. Below are Dr. and Mrs. Cole in 1984 with Sir Geoffrey Slaney, a former research fellow under Cole who became president of the Royal College of Surgeons of England.

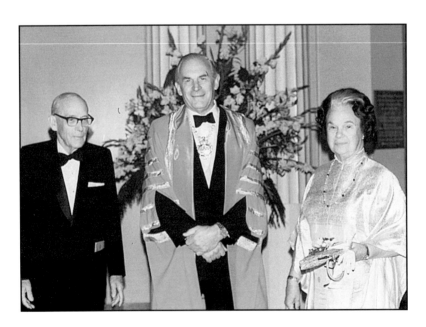

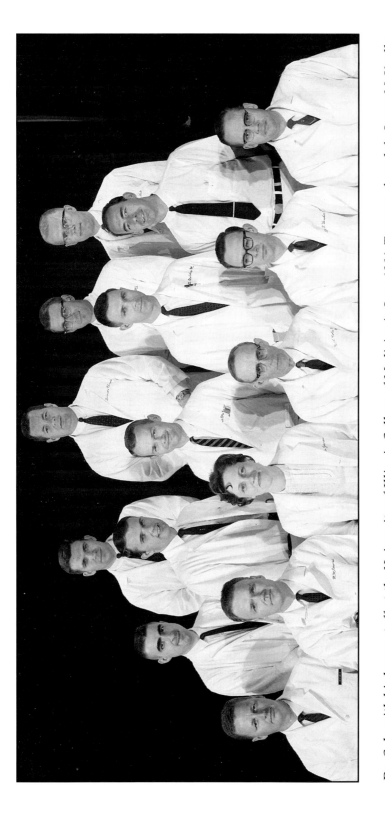

Dr. Cole with his house staff at the University of Illinois College of Medicine in June 1964. Top row, from left: Larry McKnelly, J. Anthony Brown, Mark Blum, Ardean Ediger. Middle row: James Waltz, William Jewell, Alan Graham, Elliot Goldin, John Minster. First row: Willard Smith, Marvin Romsdahl, Olga Jonasson, Warren Cole, Kenneth Vander Vennet, and Leo Robertson.

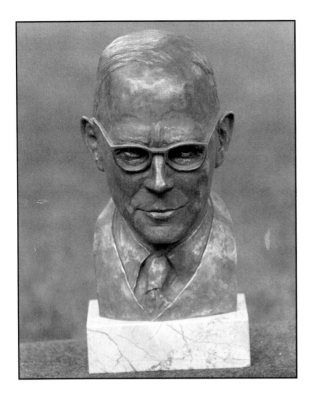

Dr. G. Howard Glassford,
a former Cole resident,
with the bust of Dr. Cole
he sculpted in 1975.

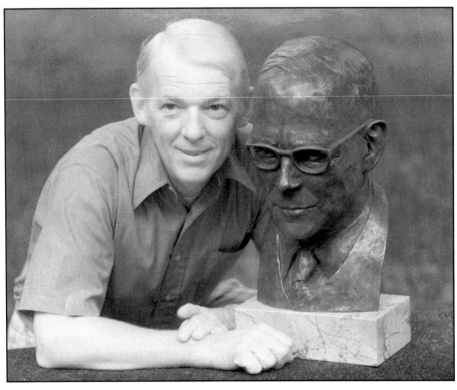

CHAPTER 12

〜

SOCIALIZED MEDICINE

F
ollowing the war, in 1947, the U.S. Department of State sent a mission made up of high-ranking scientists to the British Isles to report on the state of science and medicine in England, Scotland and Wales. The State Department gathered experts from the fields of biochemistry, chemistry, biology, physics, engineering, medicine and agriculture to spend time in Britain and report back to the United States.

Dr. Cole was asked to take part in the project as half of a two-man team sent to evaluate medicine and surgery in the United Kingdom. Dr. George Burch, head of the department of medicine at Tulane University School of Medicine in New Orleans, was the other half of the team. In early 1948, they spent three months visiting medical schools in Britain and learning all they could about medicine and surgery as practiced there. "I am not sure that I found out the exact purpose of the plan," Dr. Cole wrote in later years. "However, it was apparent we were to act as medical ambassadors to cement the friendship between the U.S. and the British.

"We were scheduled to spend two or three days each in the departments of surgery and medicine in 20 to 25 medical schools in England, Scotland and Wales. We spent most of our time discussing surgical and medical problems, although social commitments were, of course, included in our activities. Under the State Department plan, we were to interview no more than two or three members of each department, although we would meet briefly with many more.

"By following the plan, we would learn the various techniques and procedures as practiced by the members of these departments. We were not told by the State Department that our visit to the various departments was to be critical. Accordingly, we made no effort to criticize. In fact, I was amazed how little variance I found between our own methods and the British methods."

Despite the similarities, there was one major event taking place in Britain that the State Department was keenly interested in learning more about—the start-up of the National Health Service. Britain's National Health Service Act had swept through Parliament, despite opposition from the Conservative Party, and went into law in November 1946. Scheduled to begin in July 1948, just after Cole's visit, the National Health Service was designed to provide comprehensive health care for all citizens, financed by government tax revenues.

The spirit of unity and solidarity in the face of a common enemy that characterized England in World War II directly influenced public policy after the war. According to Derek Fraser, professor of English history at the University of California in Los Angeles, the English people had accepted the almost limitless sacrifices of the war effort in return for the implied promise of a "more enlightened, more open postwar society." World War II tended to reduce social distinctions. Rich and poor alike needed shelter and protection from Hitler's bombs, and the war required the combined efforts and support of the entire population. Thus the idea of universalism and the goal of a brighter future, linked with the country's war-time dependence on government to coordinate social needs, led naturally to the development of the British welfare state. Warfare opened the way to welfare.

British social planners envisioned a womb-to-tomb social security system of benefits for childbirth, widows and orphans, health care, unemployment, industrial injury, old age, and funerals, all supported by a single weekly contribution

from the citizenry. The newly elected Labour government en-
acted a package of legislative acts to accomplish those goals.
Health care was the realm of the National Health Service Act.
Once passed, the act made comprehensive health and re-
habilitation services available to all citizens through an administrative structure that involved hospitals, medical services, and local health and welfare authorities. Both
voluntary hospitals and local health authorities were na-
tionalized and put under the control of 20 regional hospital
boards appointed by the Minister of Health.

In his confidential report to the State Department, Dr.
Cole described the British health system as he found it in the
spring of 1948 and the changes that the new National Health
Service would bring. Britain already had a national health
plan before the new act went into effect, but its coverage was
uneven.

"At the present time (May 1948), about 45 percent of the
people are covered by a type of national insurance," Cole
wrote. "These people were assigned to a physician's list or
panel; the average number on one panel is perhaps slightly
over 1,000, although there may be a maximum of 2,500. The
physician is paid an annual per capita fee of 15s.6d ($3.10) for
each member of his panel. The individual on the panel is entitled to free care by the physician, although his wife and children are not. The physician is entitled to make a small charge
of $1.00 to $2.00 per visit for these members of the family. In
addition, the physician is entitled to have other private patients. All of the specialty or consultant work is done on the
basis of private practice; specialists are not assigned to a
panel."

Socialized medicine and national health insurance are issues that come up for debate regularly in the United States.
Some point to the British and Canadian systems as models to
be emulated, while others damn national health schemes as
inefficient, wasteful and antithetical to high-quality health
care. Warren Cole was clearly on the side of the critics from
the beginning.

"The new National Health Service Act going into effect
July 5th, 1948, contains many prominent changes from previous conditions, although a type of socialized medicine was

in effect before that date," he wrote in his State Department report. "The new Act states that all citizens are to enter the insurance plan; all doctors are invited to participate in it, although specialists or consultants will remain as a group obtaining a large portion of their income from private practice. The physician's income will be derived from a basic salary ($1,200 per year) and an annual per capita fee ($3.05) from each of the members of his panel.

"This phase of the Act will almost certainly depreciate the caliber of service rendered the patient. If the doctor is extremely conscientious, the service rendered the patient will not be adversely affected, but from observations on the service extended to the patient under the preexisting panel system, the outlook on service is not good, since on so many occasions the patient was not thoroughly examined but was given prescriptions of various types for complaints not well investigated. The fact that the patient is satisfied *cannot be used as a criterion* that a given system is satisfactory, since the patient may be entirely contented with a handful of highly colored pills and freedom from the inconvenience of frequent examinations."

Cole also criticized the Act because it vested so much power in one person, the Minister of Health. "The Minister of Health has practically complete authority in all matters pertaining to the Act, including a *strong* voice in the appointment of numerous committees appointed for execution of the various programs of the Act; all of these committees are directly responsible to the Minister. Such a system might work efficiently and advantageously so long as the Minister is sincere, honest and wise in the health needs of the nation. An outsider is almost certain to doubt that these conditions can be expected, particularly when changes in the ruling body are apt to take place every few years; of most importance, one would be driven to the conclusion that no one man could be sufficiently well qualified in social and medical problems to execute that power wisely."

And finally, Cole felt that the national health service would have a detrimental effect on physicians. "A close doctor-patient relationship, as cherished by most patients, almost certainly cannot exist under the provisions of the new Act, except in the care of patients by specialists in their private practice. Moreover, the Act would certainly tend to destroy initiative and desire on the part of the physician to improve himself scientifically, since most of the incentive for improvement in his scientific qualifications will have been eliminated. Of more than trivial importance is the fact that the vast majority of physicians dislike the terms of the Act. It was learned long ago that discontent among workers, regardless of the type involved, tends to depreciate the quality of service rendered."

Indeed, the British Medical Association polled its 47,000 members in January of 1948 and found that about 80 percent objected to the Act in its initial form. The Minister of Health, Aneurin Bevan, who was the architect of the Act, realized that in the end, only the doctors could make the health system work. So he set about to win the support of the high echelons of medicine by an approach designed to divide and conquer. Bevan capitalized on the historic split between the elite consultants who belonged to the Royal Colleges and the ordinary general practitioner by awarding important financial concessions to the consultants. His plan was to buy off the consultants in return for their support. (In his own words, he wanted to "stuff their mouths with gold.") Consultants were allowed to work part-time in the hospitals for higher salaries, continue private practice, and have their own beds for private patients in the hospitals without limits on the fees they could charge.

Despite these favors, however, the British Medical Association, forcefully led by Dr. Guy Dain as president and Dr. Charles Hill as secretary, persisted in its opposition to provisions of the Act that limited the free choice of physicians to practice where and how they chose. Bevan countered that doctors and patients were free to join the National Health Service or not, but he knew that the scheme would not work without sufficient numbers of doctors. The biggest fear physicians had was that they would eventually be forced into a full-time salaried position, with the salary set by the state. To offset that fear, Bevan announced in April of 1948 that salaried service would not be introduced without another act of Parliament and that most doctors would be paid solely on the basis of capitation fees.

In an article published by the *American Practitioner* magazine in October of 1948, Dr. Cole and Dr. Burch wrote of Bevan's other promises to physicians. "The Minister has assured the medical profession that every physician will be free to practice where he pleases unless there are more doctors than are needed in that area. Likewise, he has stated that all physicians will be free to choose assistants or partners. Freedom of speech has been guaranteed in professional and scientific activities. The Minister has also offered assurance that hospitals will be given the privilege of accepting or refusing new appointments to their staff. Private accommodations [for private patients] in hospitals have been promised."

Following those assurances by the Minister, opposition from the medical community dwindled rapidly. "Partly because of these concessions on the part of the Minister and partly because of fear that failure to register for participation in the Act might jeopardize their financial security, many of the physicians voting originally not to cooperate voted in the last plebiscite to participate in the Act," Cole and Burch wrote. "At a meeting of the representative body of the B.M.A. in May, the members voted 167 to 148 to accept the provisions of the Act. However, certain of the opponents are very bitterly opposed to the Act, and they declare that the fight will be carried on because the 'sign or starve' policy adopted by the government represents a breach in the promise of individual freedom of the British citizen."

After that dramatic meeting of the British Medical Association on May 28, 1948, about 18,000 physicians agreed to join the National Health Service in its first year, although some did so ruefully. By December 1948, some 21 million previously uninsured British subjects had signed on for the new health service, along with the 19 million workers who were already insured under the old plan. From the very beginning, the demand for medical services was high and costs went way beyond what anyone had anticipated, skyrocketing to more that four million pounds in the first year alone. Costs and charges for the health service escalated, and in 1951, Aneurin Bevan resigned as Minister of Health over the issue of charges.

Like many in medicine, Dr. Cole felt throughout his life

that national health insurance was a concept that would not work in the United States. No one can say what effect Cole's report on the British National Health Service actually had on long-term health policy in America. He always felt that doctors in this country would staunchly oppose the socialization of medicine.

But no matter what the political ramifications of Cole's mission to Great Britain were, there were significant social and professional benefits to his trip. The professional contacts that he established in England and Scotland led to an exchange of surgical trainees from Great Britain to the University of Illinois and other medical schools around the country. In 1953, Cole was made chairman of a committee set up by the American College of Surgeons to work with the Horse Shoe Club of Britain, a group formed in England in 1932 with the stated purpose of "fostering friendship and the exchange of medical research and clinical workers between the United States, Canada and Great Britain." Through this exchange program, a string of about 15 young British surgeons were sent to study under Cole for a year or two as research fellows at the U. of I. The program led to an interchange of knowledge between the two countries and a greater understanding of the medical problems faced by other nations.

World War II had been detrimental to Cole's research program on the home front because less outside funding was available for research that was not related to war injuries, and the war siphoned off students and faculty alike. Once the war was over, he was able to crank up his research machine again and move into new areas of study.

From the beginning of his research career at Washington University until the end of the war, Cole had concentrated on diseases of the liver, biliary tract and thyroid gland but ventured into other diseases as well. "Hence, during the years from 1928 to the end of the Second World War," wrote Dr. Loren Humphrey, a former resident of Dr. Cole and now professor of surgery at the University of Missouri Medical School in Columbia, "this surgeon's interest, while still focused a great deal on the biliary tract and the thyroid gland, expanded to other areas, such as acute peritonitis, congenital malformations of the intestinal tract, portal obstruction, pancreatitis, hepatopancreatic problems and diseases of the spleen. As can be seen from that list and a perusal of Cole's bibliography during these years, he was becoming a complete surgeon, as certainly one must to assume the chair of a major university surgical department and the responsibility of educating medical students and training young men as surgeons for the community."

"He continued during the period after the war," Dr. Humphrey observed, "to write on biliary tract diseases and various general surgical topics, such as treatment of peptic ulcer, intestinal obstruction, and lesions of the pancreas, while his articles on treating strictures of the common duct and common duct diseases had brought him recognition as one of the premier surgeons in treating these severe diseases and iatrogenic problems of the hepatobiliary tree."

In the post-war period, Dr. Cole also began research into a disease that was, and still is, one of the major killers in the world—cancer. His discoveries in the treatment of cancer would bring him international recognition, enhance his already formidable reputation for genius in research and assure his place in history as one of the surgical greats in the last half of the 20th century. It would also bring him into the eye of a controversy that severely damaged the reputation of a great university, toppled a highly respected educator from power and deluded a vast number of cancer patients.

"The cancer research was gradual," Dr. Cole said in 1989. "At the time, I was studying different phases of surgery to keep the pot boiling in all directions." In 1945, the *Rocky Mountain Medical Journal* published his very first article on cancer, titled "Carcinoma of the Colon," in which he described the results of a variety of methods used to treat colon cancer patients at the University of Illinois over an eight-year period. In 1947, he published another article on the same subject in the *Illinois Medical Journal*. There was a tumor clinic connected to the Research and Educational Hospitals at the U. of I. that afforded Dr. Cole and his staff and residents the opportunity to see and treat cancer patients. In the late 1940s, Cole looked into the effects of stilbestrol, a synthetic crystalline compound, on the treatment of various types of malignant tumors.

But even before he published any research on cancer per se, he and a colleague named Lewis Rossiter published a paper in the *Annals of Surgery* in 1944 that identified a benign lesion that might develop into cancer, which the authors classified as precancerous hyperplasia (an increase in the number of cells in a tissue or organ). "Lost in his more visible contributions is a study carried out with Lewis Rossiter," according to Dr. Humphrey. "This study was the first article to describe a precancerous benign lesion, and for this Cole should be given priority since only years later has the scientific community recognized that atypical hyperplasia is the lesion that gives women with fibrocystic disease a greater risk of developing carcinoma of the breast."

Today, of course, women are urged to examine their own breasts for lumps that might be cancerous; cancer experts know that the earlier the disease is discovered, the easier it is to treat successfully. Cole and Rossiter's description of these precancerous lesions was one of the first giant steps forward in the early detection and treatment of breast cancer. The two further collaborated on a medical text titled *The Breast*, which was published in 1944.

In 1949, Cole combined his interest in cancer with his long-term study of thyroid disease to produce a paper published in *Surgery, Gynecology & Obstetrics* on the surgical treatment of "Carcinoma of the Thyroid Gland." His co-authors were Dr. Danely Slaughter, director of the tumor clinic at the University of Illinois, and Dr. J.D. Majarakis, who was working on a master of science degree in surgery under Dr. Cole. In the same year, Cole published a book on general surgery called *Operative Technic*. The book was a compilation of chapters written by experts in various aspects of surgery, all edited by Cole.

Cole was doing other important research at the time as well, notably an animal study to determine the toxic factors in blood resulting from burns, but it was his work in cancer and his position as full-time head of surgery that put him in the vortex of a maelstrom that was just beginning to form in the late 1940s at the University of Illinois. Following the war, returning soldiers began to flood the halls of university and medical schools all over the country, and Illinois was no exception. Undergraduate enrollment at Illinois more than doubled between 1945 and 1946, and the College of Medicine had to reject more than 450 applicants because its facilities were not equipped to accommodate the influx of students. Still, the 167 applicants it did accept in 1946 made it once again one of the largest medical schools in the country.

The university's new president, George D. Stoddard, created a new post at the medical center in Chicago, that of Vice-President of the University in Charge of the Chicago Professional Colleges of Medicine, Dentistry and Pharmacy. The main campus of the University of Illinois is in Urbana, some 120 miles south of Chicago, and so the Chicago campus, consisting of the professional colleges, needed an administrative head on site. Previously, the dean of the College of Medicine had acted as administrative head, but the deans of the other professional colleges began to complain.

In 1946, Stoddard appointed Andrew C. Ivy to the position. Five years later, the names of these two administrators would become inextricably linked in one of the most scandalous and bizarre incidents in the history of 20th century medicine. At the time, however, Ivy seemed an excellent choice for the new post. Author of several books and hundreds of scientific papers, he was head of the division of physiology and pharmacology at Northwestern University in Chicago, where he had spent the past 20 years. During World War II, he founded and was director of the Naval Medical Research Institute, and after the war, he acted as a consultant on medical ethics before the Nuremburg Tribunal on War Crimes. The medical faculty wanted Ivy to join the university in order to strengthen its research program. The faculty initially suggested the vice-president's position as a inducement to get Ivy.

And so in 1946, Dr. Andrew C. Ivy joined the faculty of the University of Illinois as distinguished professor of physiology, head of the department of clinical science and vice-president of the university. His only superior in administration was President Stoddard. From the time of his appointment until 1951, Ivy proved to be a respected research scientist in an environment that placed a premium on research and a first-rate fund raiser at a state-run university that desperately needed to enlarge its aging facilities.

Then in 1951, Ivy called a conference on new cancer research that would raise the hopes of cancer patients everywhere and weaken the foundations of scientific inquiry for the next 15 years.

CHAPTER **13**

ক্ষ

KREBIOZEN—THE SCANDAL THAT WOULD NOT DIE

D r. Andrew C. Ivy, vice-president of the University of Illinois in charge of the Chicago professional colleges, had a theory that he believed would lead to a cure for cancer. His idea, which he first articulated in 1917 when he was 24 years old, was that humans and animals who do not have cancer must have a anti-cancer substance in their tissue and blood that is capable of resisting the disease.

In 1949, a mysterious Yugoslavian physician named Stevan Durovic came to him with a natural substance, extracted from a horse, that Durovic claimed would shrink malignant tumors. Ivy shared Durovic's enthusiasm for the substance and eagerly supported an 18-month clinical investigation.

In March of 1951, Dr. Warren Cole received a letter from Dr. Andrew Ivy that contained a startling announcement. The letter, dated March 16, read as follows:

> During the past 18 months Doctor Stevan Durovic of Yugoslavia, Doctors L. R. Krasno, W. F. P. Phillips, John F. Pick, Mr. L. E. Grubgeld, and I have been investigating the effectiveness of a substance called 'Krebiozen' on malignant tumors.
>
> The substance was discovered by Doctor Durovic.

The other persons mentioned have been concerned only in testing it for toxicity and for its promise in the management of patients with cancer.

The substance is extracted by a chemical process from the blood serum of a horse several weeks after the horse has been injected with a substance which, as is commonly stated, 'stimulates' the reticuloendothelial system.

Up to January 1, 1951, 22 patients have been treated and observed long enough for us to believe that a preliminary report of our observations to a limited group of physicians and a group of lay persons, who have been connected in some way with our study, is appropriate and warranted.

It is believed that we have observed favorable results in 20 of the 22 patients, and we are positive that the substance is *per se* essentially non-toxic in man and animals, and produces *per se* no undesirable side reactions. In view of the pathological anatomy of cancer, we have used the substance with caution in patients with internal cancer.

It is my opinion that the substance merits a thorough clinical study and investigation, since I believe it possesses much promise in the management of the cancer patient.

With this idea in mind several physicians, who direct much attention to the management of cancer patients, are being invited to a meeting at which our observations will be presented and a document, which provides our observations in considerable detail, will be distributed.

You are cordially invited to attend the meeting which will be held at the Drake Hotel (Chicago) in the French Room on Monday, March 26th at 3:00 p.m. The meeting should be completed by 5:00 p.m.

After the meeting we should like for you to direct a letter to me if you would like to obtain some of the material with the understanding that you will provide us with a brief synopsis of your observations relative to the use of the material.

Hoping that it will be possible for you to attend, I am

Yours sincerely,
A. C. Ivy, Ph.D., M.D.

The invitation was odd in a number of ways. First, Ivy was ready to spring his news at a public meeting without having published his research in any of the medical journals and without having discussed his research with either Dr. Cole, who was at that time involved in cancer studies, or Dr. Danely Slaughter, head of the tumor clinic at the University of Illinois. Second, Ivy's invitation neglected to mention that the Drake Hotel meeting was being held not only for "physicians who direct much attention to the management of cancer patients" but also for drug company executives, politicians, prominent businessmen and newspaper reporters.

Ivy proved to be a shrewd manipulator of the media and a smooth politico. As vice-president of a state-funded university, he had to be savvy in the ways of state politics, and as the top administrator at a public university medical center, he had to be polished at public relations. Along with Dr. Cole, those who attended Ivy's meeting were David Rockefeller, Senator Everett Dirksen, Chicago Mayor Martin Kennelly, State's Attorney John Boyle, pharmaceutical executive J. J. Lilly, and Park Livingston, president of the board of trustees of the University of Illinois. And perhaps most important, reporters from the Chicago dailies were there, eager for a story.

The brochure that Ivy handed out at the swank Drake Hotel in March of 1951 described the hypothesis driving Krebiozen research. "Doctor Durovic has worked on the basis of the following hypothesis: Every living cell contains a regulator of its proliferative activity, which is also influenced by its surrounding environment. This regulator is called 'Krebiozen.' It controls the permeability of the cell or the enzyme systems of the cell, so that in its absence or deficiency, anaerobic oxidation and acidity of the cells is increased and uncontrolled growth occurs.

"It was further hypothesized that Krebiozen is present especially in the reticuloendothelial cells, which, as is well known, react to various stimuli. When these cells are properly stimulated, Krebiozen, which is not present in the blood under normal conditions, is released and can be extracted from the blood plasma.

"Finally, Doctor Durovic hypothesized that if Krebiozen is supplied, the cells in early stages of malignancy will be normalized and those in advanced stages of malignancy will be killed or damaged and removed by phagocytosis."

Durovic's hypothesis seemed to confirm Ivy's theory that healthy humans and animals have a natural anti-cancer substance in their blood. Perhaps that explains Ivy's whole-hearted endorsement of Durovic and Krebiozen. After all, Ivy was a respected research scientist and noted administrator. He had even worked with the National Cancer Institute to establish guidelines for testing potential anti-cancer drugs. It is doubtful that Durovic would have gotten any attention for his enigmatic substance if Ivy had not placed his name and reputation on the line to back widespread clinical trials of Krebiozen, which he did at the Drake Hotel meeting.

The 106-page brochure that Ivy handed out described how Krebiozen was produced: "According to the hypothesis, Doctor Durovic stimulated the reticuloendothelial system of the horse and separated from the serum by a chemical process the Krebiozen in a pure or almost pure state. The product obtained is a white powder which is soluble in water, mineral oil, and most organic solvents. When the aqueous solution is kept in ampules, a precipitate may form in some ampules after six months. For this reason a solution in paraffin oil (#9) has been used as a rule in treating patients. The ampules after filling and sealing are autoclaved at 15 pounds pressure for 20 minutes. Doctor Durovic has found that the solution in mineral oil or olive oil is still active in ampules after 2 years."

Ivy claimed that Krebiozen halted tumor growth—and in some cases even melted tumors away—and that it enhanced the quality of life by easing the pain, aiding appetite, allowing patients to sleep better, lengthening life and imparting a sense of well-being. The brochure contained glossy photographs of cancerous tissue and tumors being measured to show shrinkage, along with the words of 22 patients telling how they were near death until they took Krebiozen; some were present at the conference to offer further testament to the drug's power.

Despite the unusual way that the discovery of Krebiozen was announced, the press ate the news up and spit it out in headlines across the nation and around the world. According to Patricia Spain Ward, campus historian at the University of Illinois in Chicago, "Journalists present at the fateful meeting at the Drake Hotel quickly supplied the word 'cure' which Ivy had studiously avoided."

Because Ivy had not consulted anyone at the U. of I. prior to his announcement, the newspaper reports "struck the College of Medicine like a thunderbolt," Ward wrote. "In Chicago and downstate, the University was totally unprepared for the ensuing deluge of telephone calls, telegrams, cablegrams, and letters that poured in from physicians—and from desperate cancer patients and their families."

But while the press and the public were lured into a belief in the power of Krebiozen, the medical community was not nearly so enamored. On May 15, 1951, an editorial appeared in the learned *Proceedings of the Institute of Medicine*, which read in part:

"Medical science has established procedures and standards of reporting progress of experimental and clinical results. The announcement in Chicago, March 26, 1951, of Krebiozen, described as an 'important step' toward a final goal of chemotherapy of cancer, ignored these procedures and standards. There was no publication in a medical or scientific journal; there was no presentation made before a learned society. Instead, Krebiozen was announced to a mixed group of physicians, medical educators, public officials, and representatives of the press. The information provided on this unusual occasion met few of the accepted criteria of medical reporting. One of the essentials when a new biological agent is presented is a clear account of the technic of its preparation or isolation and, when possible, an exact and complete description of its composition. No such information was provided as to Krebiozen, except that it was separated from the serum of a horse after 'stimulation' of its reticuloendothelial cells. Its method of preparation and its composition are expressly stated to be secret. The booklet distributed at this meeting, which purported to give clinical details on 22 cases, was gravely deficient for the purposes of evaluation."

Patricia Ward has an explanation for why Ivy bypassed all the conventional medical means of unveiling new research: "Ivy later explained that he had chosen this time and manner to announce Krebiozen because [Illinois Senator Paul] Douglas, long a close friend, had said Ivy must quickly produce some dramatic public demonstration of Krebiozen's potential so that Douglas could persuade Congress to grant citizenship to the Durovics [Stevan and his brother Marco], whose visas would soon expire." After the news of Krebiozen hit the public press, Senator Douglas easily passed a special act of Congress that granted citizenship to the Durovics.

The Durovics had escaped Yugoslavia during World War II and fled to Argentina under Vatican visas. In Buenos Aires, the brothers set up the Duga Biological Institute where Stevan allegedly did his initial research on Krebiozen and developed an anti-hypertensive drug he called Cositerin. After the Durovics arrived in Chicago in 1949, Stevan went to faculty researchers at Northwestern University to interest them in Cositerin, but subsequent tests revealed it was ineffective in reducing hypertension in dogs. Then Stevan went to Ivy at the University of Illinois with his claims for Krebiozen, which some believe was Cositerin under a new name.

Following the announcement to the world of Krebiozen's wonders, the drug's promoters formed a non-profit foundation, the Krebiozen Research Foundation, and made Ivy its president. The foundation's stated purpose was "to foster research on Krebiozen and to investigate other human ills, and to remove any reason for the suspicion of a primary commercial motivation in the investigation of Krebiozen." Meanwhile, however, the Durovics, backed by Alberto Barreira, a millionaire Argentine landowner and retired officer of the Argentine air force, set up a pharmaceutical operation to produce the drug.

While Ivy and his cohorts continued testing Krebiozen on cancer patients through their research foundation, the American Medical Association began an independent evaluation of the substance and Ivy's claims for it. The results were published in the *Journal of the American Medical Association* on October 27, 1951, under the title "Status Report on Krebiozen." Four cancer specialists around the country used Krebiozen to treat 100 patients following the protocols established by Ivy and Durovic. They found that Krebiozen had no effect.

In response to the *JAMA* article, the president of the University of Illinois, George Stoddard, called for a meeting with medical faculty members to decide what to do about Ivy and his research. Dr. Cole could not attend that meeting but wrote to Stoddard. The letter, dated November 1, 1951, spelled out his recommendations for action:

"In the first place, I look upon the Krebiozen problem primarily from the standpoint of the effect upon the University. True enough, I have always had the greatest admiration for Dr. Ivy, and appreciate the multiplicity of things he has done for the University and the medical profession. However, I think that University interests should supersede that of any one individual.

"You are, no doubt, aware of the Council meeting of the Chicago Medical Society early this month (November 12th), at which time a decision will be reached regarding infringement by Dr. Ivy on rules and regulations of the Medical Society. Frankly, I do not know what this decision will be. However, the feeling is strong enough in the Council itself to make it obvious that the verdict will not be less than censure. It is possible that the vote might be expulsion for one year, or longer. There might be one advantage in holding off any University decision until the Medical Society verdict is known, particularly if the verdict were expulsion. Counterbalancing this reaction is the reaction of the public at large, which is a great admirer of Dr. Ivy. I think we should also include the members of the State Legislature in this group. However, if Dr. Ivy did resign shortly after the Medical Society verdict (particularly if it were for expulsion), we would presumably not want to make a University verdict shortly thereafter lest it appear that University opinion was being influenced by the Medical Society verdict. Proper delay in the University verdict would obviate this impression.

"Accordingly, I personally do not have a concrete idea on a solution to the problem at the present time. If Dr. Ivy should offer his resignation it would appear entirely safe to me to postpone action for a short time until we could observe further reaction from the recent report in the *Journal of the American Medical Association*, the Chicago Medical Society verdict, etc. However, it is very true that if public opinion from the medical profession should accentuate sharply, there might be an urgent indication for action from the University."

Stoddard took Cole's advice and adopted a wait-and-see attitude. The Chicago Medical Society did indeed censure Dr. Ivy and suspended him for three months, as of November 12. But Ivy did not resign from the university. His defense against the AMA report was that it was not based on controlled clinical trials, but neither were his own conclusions about the effectiveness of the drug. The university's board of trustees met in executive session on November 23. Krebiozen had become a time bomb, and the trustees were trying to defuse it before it exploded in their faces.

In his 1981 autobiography *The Pursuit of Education*, George Stoddard wrote, "I felt that the time had come for the University of Illinois to conduct its own inquiries and come to its own conclusions regarding the nature and the clinical efficacy of Krebiozen." At the November 23 meeting, Stoddard and the trustees decided to try to validate the effects of Krebiozen on cancer patients and make their findings known to the public. President Stoddard subsequently appointed a research validation committee headed by Warren Cole to evaluate Ivy's clinical records. Beginning January 1, 1952, the board of trustees granted Ivy a two-month leave of absence from his post as vice-president to gather information for the committee, which became known as the Cole committee.

The Cole committee was composed of some big-wigs in academic cancer research: N.C. Gilbert, professor emeritus of medicine at Northwestern University; Fred Hodges, professor and chairman of the department of roentgenology at the University of Michigan; Robert Keeton, professor emeritus of medicine at the University of Illinois; Paul Steiner, professor of pathology at the University of Chicago; and

Owen Wangensteen, surgeon in chief at the University Hospital of the University of Minnesota.

"After an unavoidable delay," Stoddard reported to the trustees in 1952, "Dr. Ivy submitted to the Research Validation Committee on June 13, 1952, his report on the available cases of cancer patients that had received Krebiozen treatment. This report was in two volumes consisting of over 500 pages. Dr. Cole's committee proceeded to examine these reports and analyses and to interview Dr. Ivy and some of his associates concerning the clinical observations."

After Ivy submitted his data, the Cole committee met on June 29, July 6, and August 4, and then reported its findings to Stoddard on September 10, 1952. "On June 29th, our Committee devoted three to four hours to case reports and patient demonstrations by Dr. Ivy and his associates, and to personal discussion with Dr. Ivy," the committee said in a later statement (dated June 24, 1953). "On July 6th our Committee devoted two or three hours to a presentation by Dr. Pomeroy of experiences with Krebiozen under the direction of Dr. Reiman at Lankenau Hospital, Philadelphia, Pa."

In its report to Stoddard, the committee concluded that "it is our belief that Krebiozen has no curative value in the treatment of cancer."

Ironically, the committee was never able to determine the chemical nature of Krebiozen because Ivy told the members it was unavailable for examination. "The white powder mentioned in Dr. Ivy's report was not demonstrated to our Committee," according to its 1953 statement. "Our Committee was told by Dr. Ivy that none of the material was available because it had all been put into solution in mineral oil. If attempts should be made to extract Krebiozen from the mineral oil in which it was suspended, control extraction of the same oil would be needed, and the yield would be so small, because of the tiny amount of Krebiozen placed in solution, that concrete proof would have to be offered for identity of any substance extracted, since other substances also might be extracted."

The committee recommended to Stoddard that Krebiozen should be manufactured under close supervision following Durovic's formula. "In our opinion," the committee's report stated, "it would be inconclusive if not futile to conduct further clinical investigation unless it is first possible to dispel the mystery which surrounds the nature of the material. In default of this step no further consideration should be given to the problem."

Stoddard appointed another committee to try to determine just what Krebiozen was, but the Durovics continually evaded every attempt to force them to reveal the formulation of the substance. That committee reported: "Letters transmitted by Dr. Ivy and received by the chairman on November 11, 1952, stated that the originators of the preparation are unwilling to furnish materials and will not provide full technical information for the use of the committee within a reasonable time."

In response to the Durovics' refusals, Stoddard banned all further clinical research on Krebiozen at the University of Illinois. The president decreed "that there be no allowance of time, funds, space, equipment, patients or printing in behalf of any staff member of the University of Illinois for the clinical utilization of Krebiozen, and that every effort be made to dissociate Krebiozen from research or service programs. This action would be consistent with the major recommendations of the Cole Committee in which I have full confidence; it would, I believe, merit the support of all medical men familiar with these events." Furthermore, on November 29, 1952, Stoddard urged the board of trustees to abolish the vice-president's job held by Ivy to help resolve the Krebiozen controversy. Ivy was clearly becoming an embarrassment to the university. The board merely granted Ivy a leave of absence for six months.

The response of the medical faculty and the board of trustees of the University of Illinois to Stoddard's actions reflected the divided passions that Ivy inflamed. On one side were those who saw him as a fraud and a disgrace to the medical profession. On the other were those who viewed him as the beset-upon champion of a drug that could potentially have untold benefits for cancer patients. At its meeting on November 21, the medical faculty was asked to vote on two statements. The first one said:

"The Executive Committee of the Faculty of the College

of Medicine regrets the conduct and presentation of the research on Krebiozen and the continued interest of the Vice President in its possible anti-cancer effect in the face of competent scientific findings (including those of our Tumor Clinic) to the contrary. The Committee further regrets the loss of prestige which the office of the Vice President has incurred with the medical profession and is distressed by the confusion engendered in the minds of the faculty and students relative to research and teaching standards of the College of Medicine."

The second statement read in part: "Whereas, we believe that the matter at stake is far more important than the substance Krebiozen, its value or lack of value. The ultimatum which we understand to be contemplated is rather a *precedent*, which might end for every one of us a tradition of freedom of research within a great university. This could happen to any one of us. At stake is the future of any new idea, of any new therapeutic agent in the process of development, not for individual gain but for the good of mankind."

The faculty members defeated the second resolution by a vote of 95 to 58, and added support for Stoddard to the first: "The Executive Committee of the Faculty of the College of Medicine commends the President of the University for his stand on the Krebiozen problem." And so, in the end, the medical faculty backed Stoddard's action.

Ivy defended himself in a statement to the faculty that said: "Believe me, after the first disparaging reports and comments on the use of this material came to my attention, it would have been easier for me to disassociate promptly myself from this research. Many of my friends and associates from all over the world advised me to do just this. However, had I done this at that time, without, in my judgment, exhaustively and thoroughly studying the response of all types of tumors to this substance, I think that I would have betrayed those unfortunate human beings afflicted with cancer, who put their trust and hope in this material." Ivy further cited one of the Cole committee's conclusions that "on the basis of the evidence submitted we cannot state that it is entirely devoid of biological activity." He used this statement as justification for continued study of Krebiozen.

At the same time, in a dramatic move, the dean of the College of Medicine, Dr. Stanley Olson, who reported directly to Ivy, announced his resignation, effective January 1, 1953. He cited "basic differences of opinion between Doctor Ivy and myself" as the reason. But no matter what actions his opponents took, as Dr. Cole had indicated to President Stoddard early on, Ivy had powerful friends and supporters in the state legislature and on the university's board of trustees who continued to tolerate Ivy's methods.

The controversy became a circus when Ivy alleged that Stoddard conspired with the American Medical Association and the Chicago Medical Society to have him ousted as vice-president of the university over the Krebiozen affair. Incredibly, the Illinois state legislature convened a special committee to investigate the whole Krebiozen matter in early 1953.

One of the most bizarre charges to come out of those hearings was made by Alberto Barreira, the Argentine millionaire who was backing the Durovics. Barreira testified that the treasurer of the American Medical Association, Dr. Josiah Moore, had asked his help in 1951 to force the Durovics to sell distribution rights to Krebiozen to business friends of Moore. Ivy maintained throughout the committee's hearings and afterwards that some in organized medicine conspired to suppress Krebiozen and to steal the secret of the drug for their own profit.

In another outlandish turn to this story, while the legislative hearings were still going on, the board of trustees of the University of Illinois, at a midnight meeting on July 24, 1953, voted to force the resignation of the university's president, George Stoddard, saying it had lost confidence in his administration. Ivy was allowed to stay on the faculty of the College of Medicine, but the trustees refused to reinstate him as vice-president after his leave of absence ran out. Ironically, the legislative committee eventually concluded that both Dr. Ivy and Dr. Durovic were "men of good character" and that neither Dr. Stoddard nor the AMA had conspired against Ivy.

Stoddard moved to Princeton, New Jersey, where he wrote a book about Ivy and Krebiozen, originally titled

"Krebiozen": The Great Cancer Hoax. But Ivy won a court injunction against the publisher, Boston's Beacon Press, and Stoddard's book became, as Patricia Ward noted, the first book ever banned in Boston *before* it was published. The Massachusetts Supreme Court later overturned the injunction and the book was published in 1955 under a revised title, *"Krebiozen": The Great Cancer Mystery.* After it was published, Ivy persisted in his feud with Stoddard, who by then had become chancellor of New York University, and he filed a libel suit against his former boss, asking $360,000 in damages. The case turned out to be the longest in the history of the U.S. District Court for Northern Illinois and one of the longest libel suits on record—11 years. After some initial reading of the book aloud to the jury, the judge postponed the trial until the nature of Krebiozen could be determined. It was not until June 10, 1966, that the suit was dismissed with prejudice when Stoddard signed a statement saying he did not intend to libel Ivy.

In the meantime, Ivy and the Durovics continued dispensing their mysterious substance through the Krebiozen Research Foundation and in 1954 began asking donations for the drug ranging up to $9.50 per dose. Some patients were taking up to 20 doses a week. The drug was raking in huge sums of money, perhaps millions. Ivy defended the profit by saying that the Durovics had invested over a million dollars to develop the anti-cancer elixir. Throughout all the ballyhoo over the drug, an estimated 5,000 patients eagerly took injections of the preparation because they were solemnly convinced that it kept them alive. Some of them even picketed the Kennedy White House in 1963 to protest government action against what they called their lifeline.

Even though Stevan Durovic stealthily evaded all attempts at analyzing Krebiozen, the federal government allowed him to continue dispensing the substance because under rules of the Food and Drug Administration then in force, a drug manufacturer could distribute an experimental product as long as he could prove that the medicine was not toxic. But after another drug scandal, the thalidomide disaster, the FDA laws were tightened. In 1963, the Kefauver-Harris amendments to FDA law resulted from an investigation by

Senator Estes Kefauver into the drug industry after it was found that when pregnant women took thalidomide, a sleeping pill, their babies were often born deformed.

Under the new regulations, the FDA finally analyzed Krebiozen in 1964 and found that it contained nothing more than creatine, a common amino acid derivative "plentifully available from meat in the ordinary diet...and a normal constituent of the human body." Furthermore, the FDA declared that its samplings of the Krebiozen shipped prior to 1960 revealed nothing but mineral oil. Commented Dr. T. Philip Waalkes, who was at the time associate director of the National Cancer Institute: "It is impossible to conceive that creatine...could be of any value in treating cancer."

Illinois Senator Paul Douglas' office issued a report denouncing the FDA findings as false. Stevan Durovic responded by saying, "The FDA's plan, of course, is to harass us to such an extent that we will abandon Krebiozen. I will never do that. I believe in it. It helps patients. Krebiozen represents 33 years of my life's work. I hope we can get the help to win this fight. I believe we will win—because of the power of human justice." Dr. Ivy told a reporter, "I'm going to keep going. I'm going to continue my work. This isn't Russia. Here the creative scientist is free."

But the federal government was closing in. In November of 1964, a grand jury in Chicago indicted Ivy and the Durovics on 49 counts of failing to comply with provisions of the new FDA regulations. In a desperate move, Ivy went to the courts to enjoin Attorney General Nicholas Katzenbach from bringing him to trial on criminal charges. He was denied this action a week before his criminal trial was due to start in April of 1965. After a lengthy trial, the defendants were acquitted of all charges. The IRS soon went after the Durovics for $815,000 in back taxes and indicted the brothers on charges of tax evasion. Stevan escaped to Switzerland, never to return to the United States, and Marco contested the government's case. He lived out his life in a wealthy suburb of Chicago.

Andrew Ivy remains the chief mystery in the Krebiozen affair. He stayed on the faculty of the University of Illinois until 1962 when he retired. He then continued doing research from an office provided him by Roosevelt University in downtown Chicago. After his criminal trial, he gave up his efforts on behalf of Krebiozen but took up a new investigation—of a substance called Carcalon, derived from the blood serum of cattle, which Ivy believed could aid the body's natural defenses against cancer. Ivy died in 1978.

The major question surrounding Ivy is why he so doggedly backed the Durovics and risked his reputation on an unproven substance. "Without Ivy, there would have been no Krebiozen," said Dr. George Wakerlin, who was on the medical faculty at the University of Illinois in 1951. "After all, Doctor Ivy was no cancer quack. The medical community at first simply refused to believe that he would lend his name to an apparently worthless drug."

Some say he truly believed that the cancer patients he treated were being helped by the drug, although he certainly should have known that since all of his patients were terminal cancer patients and were being treated by other means as well—surgery, radiation therapy and chemotherapy—any improvements in their health could be due to a number of reasons.

Others look at greed as the motive. But while it is likely that the Durovics profited handsomely from Krebiozen, there is little evidence that Ivy's pockets were lined by profits from the drug.

Some of his former colleagues point to blind ambition as the cause of his downfall. "Ivy had two or three crucial weak spots," said Dr. Warren Cole in an interview in 1989. "Number one was a desire to win the Nobel Prize, and that's what ruined him. He also failed to realize that cancer patients will respond favorably to any kind of care their physician gives them. I remember that he invited me to his office early in the game to convince me of the value of Krebiozen. He pulled out a book full of statements from patients saying, invariably, that they felt better after treatment. He concluded that they were getting better from the treatment. In reality the patients were converting hope into a feeling of improvement."

Cole and his research validation committee have been criticized for being too lenient on Dr. Ivy in their report. "We were asked to study the cases and see if the cure was real,"

Cole said. "We were not told to punish Dr. Ivy. There were those who wanted us to say 'You're a damned liar,' but that was not our business." The committee's report was further criticized for concluding that "on the basis of evidence submitted we cannot state that it is entirely devoid of biological activity." But in its follow-up statement in June of 1953, the committee clarified its intent: "It was then and still is the considered opinion of our Committee that neither the written report of Dr. Ivy nor the evidence in patients shown by Dr. Ivy and his group before our Committee proved that Krebiozen had any favorable biological activity in cancer."

Although the University of Illinois was shaken to its research foundations by the cruel hoax known as Krebiozen, Dr. Cole returned to his own research on cancer and was soon to reveal discoveries that would make a real difference for cancer patients for generations to come.

CHAPTER 14

𝕫𝕒

COMBATING CANCER

I n the early part of the 20th century, cancer was a disease that was only talked about in whispers. It was thought to be contagious and considered a disgrace to the patient's family. But by the time Krebiozen came along in the 1950s, medical research had pointed to genetic and environmental causes of cancer, and the public had become hungry for information about symptoms and early detection as a means of prevention.

The U.S. government began keeping statistics on the incidence of cancer in the population in the early 1930s. By 1950, it was clear that cancer was steadily on the rise, and in fact, it had become the number two killer in our society. In 1900, influenza and tuberculosis topped the list of deadly diseases in the United States; by 1950, they were supplanted by heart disease and cancer. Among the reasons for the increase in cancer were the overall growth of the population, more accurate diagnosis, an increase in life expectancy so that more people were reaching ages at which cancer strikes more frequently, and the growth in technology, which resulted in greater exposure to cancer-causing chemicals and pollutants.

Surgery was by far the most common method of treating cancer. Surgical removal of internal cancers became possible in the 19th century after the introduction of anesthesia and aseptic techniques. Every part of the human anatomy, even the brain, became accessible to the surgeon's scalpel in the 20th century due to advances in surgical technique and the use of blood transfusions and antibiotics. Halsted perfected the radical mastectomy for breast cancer in the early 20th century, Harvey Cushing developed triumphant operations to remove tumors of the brain around 1910, and Evarts Graham succeeded in the first removal of a cancerous lung in 1933.

X-ray therapy was little used to treat cancer prior to 1920, except for superficial skin cancers. However, with advances in x-ray equipment and an understanding of how to measure doses of radiation and grade tumors according to their susceptibility to radiation came increasing use of x-ray treatment for cancer.

In the 1950s, chemotherapy as a tool against cancer was still in an evolutionary stage. It was not until after World War II that nitrogen mustards were declassified from the federal government's top-secret list and the results of wartime research published. Sulfur mustard, or mustard gas, was used in combat in World War I, and its toxic effects on lymphoid tissue led to research on nitrogen mustards as anti-cancer agents. These gases became the first chemotherapeutic agents to be widely used against lymphoid tumors and later as immunosuppressive agents as well.

A major advance in the fight against cancer during the war years was the development, by Dr. George N. Papanicolaou, of a diagnostic procedure that allowed examination under a microscope of cells shed by a tumor, a procedure popularly known as the Pap smear. In 1943, Papanicolaou and Herbert Trout published their classic monograph, "Diagnosis of Uterine Cancer by the Vaginal Smear."

Following World War II, Dr. Cole began a series of studies of patients who underwent operations for cancer of the colon at the University of Illinois Hospitals. He began to document the high incidence of new colon and rectal tumors that appeared after patients had a primary operation for cancer. He concluded that the operation itself was spreading deadly tumor cells. In an article published in the July 1951 issue of *The American Surgeon*, the same year that Ivy made his initial announcement about Krebiozen, Dr. Cole first mentioned in print what was to become a major contribution to the care of cancer patients:

"At the present time the author is deeply concerned over the possibility that we may be negligent in the prevention of the relatively frequent recurrences of tumor at the stoma when anterior resection for carcinoma of the rectum and rectosigmoid is performed. A serious defect in our technic exists. For example, it is well known from examination of rectal secretions in patients with carcinoma of the rectum and sigmoid that cancer cells (presumably alive) are found in the lumen many inches distal to the lesion. Yet when we cut across the lumen of the bowel distal to the lesion, we do little or nothing to prevent transplantation of these desquamated cells from the lumen into the cut section of the bowel at the anastomotic site.

"Seldom indeed does a recurrence develop in the terminal end of a colostomy, even though the bowel is often transected no more than 8 to 10 cm. from the upper edge of the tumor, which is removed by the Miles technic along with all of the distal rectum. Since recurrence is found so rarely in the end of the colostomy proximal to an excised cancer, and since lymphatic drainage is proximally, and rarely travels more than three or four cm. distally from the tumor, there appears to be circumstantial evidence that we may be seeding cells recently desquamated or dislodged by our manipulation, from the tumor, into the cut end of the remaining bowel at the site of the anastomosis.

"Thorough irrigation of the distal segment of the rectum after ligature of the bowel between the tumor and proposed site of anastomosis, along with instillation of certain chemicals, are factors which deserve consideration in the prevention of possible seeding from desquamated cells. A study of these factors is being made in our clinic at the present time."

In layman's terms, what Cole was telling his surgical colleagues was that when the surgeon cut into the colon and removed a cancerous tumor, he or she was probably shedding live cancer cells into the colon and rectum, especially at the place where the cut was made. Furthermore, Cole was recommending that anti-cancer chemicals be used to kill the seeded cancer cells at the time of the operation.

As *The American Surgeon* article indicated, Cole and his research team continued their studies into the problem. In 1952, Cole published the first in a series of scientific reports to prove his hypothesis that the very handling of a tumor during an operation to remove it resulted in shedding of live cancer cells inside the patient. At the same time, he studied ways of preventing the seeding or implantation of loose cancer cells.

"My colleagues and I have gone over records at Illinois Research Hospital," Cole wrote for the *Archives of Surgery* in 1952, "and find that in 55 consecutive patients having local resection for carcinoma of the colon and proximal portion of the rectum over a five-year period between 1944 and 1950 (exclusive of Miles operations), there was an incidence of local recurrence equal to 16%. In this group of nine recurrences, six occurred at the suture line, constituting an incidence of 10.9% in which recurrence by implantation was possible."

In the introduction to this report, Cole observed: "It is obvious that there is enough manipulation of the tumor during the resection to result in desquamation [shedding] of numerous cancer cells from the primary lesion. Moreover, we now know with the aid of the Papanicolaou stain that cancer cells desquamate profusely from ulcerating tumors. Although it is unlikely that these desquamated cells would become implanted on normal mucosa, it may be assumed that they might become implanted on open wounds or ulcerated areas and grow. There is ample evidence that cancer cells can be implanted in breast wounds during radical mastectomy, and in wounds following many other types of radical operation for cancer. If implantation can occur in certain types of operation, it is logical to assume it might take place in others."

The statement was classic Cole. As he proved in his studies on cholecystography, his genius lay in simple observation and cold logic—and the dogged pursuit of a solution to the problem. In the *Archives of Surgery* paper, Cole raised the possibility of using chemotherapy to kill the cells that shed from the tumor. "We have not used any chemicals in our attempt to destroy loose cancer cells," he wrote, "but if we did, we should probably choose a weak solution of iodine tincture."

His surgical approach to stopping the further spread of cancer cells after a bowel operation was to tie off the colon several centimeters before and behind the site of the tumor prior to handling the tumor, then to clamp the colon during the operation. "As the diseased bowel is being resected, clamps are applied to the colon proximally and distally, and each segment is irrigated thoroughly with distilled water before anastomosis [suturing together the cut ends of the colon] is performed. After the irrigation, a small segment is resected from either end to eliminate the possibility that cells may have been trapped in the wall at the site of application of the clamp."

In 1954, Cole and his research colleagues published two articles in the *Journal of the American Medical Association* reporting further studies of surgery for colon cancer and the spread of malignant cells. In one, they took Pap smears of the lining of the colon to determine the extent of cell spread. "To explore the possibility of recurrent carcinoma of the bowel arising from tumor cells lying free in the lumen of the colon and becoming implanted by the suturing needle or on cut surfaces at lines of anastomosis, Papanicolaou smear preparations of mucus from the lining surface of colon specimens removed for carcinoma were examined. Apparently well-preserved and possibly viable malignant cells were present in smears of 42% of the proximal ends and 65% of the distal ends of the resected colons at average distances from the tumors of 21 cm. and 10 cm., respectively. Such cells were found as far as 35 cm. from the tumor in one instance and in more than half of the smears taken at a distance commonly considered safe for resection (10 to 15 cm.). This strongly suggests that occasional implantation and growth of these free cells may be responsible for recurrences."

Now that Cole was reasonably certain that malignant cancer cells are set free during operation, he had to face the problem of how to destroy them. "It was pretty easy to tell the benign cells from the malignant cells," said Dr. Elizabeth McGrew, a co-author of one of the *JAMA* papers and a pathologist and cytologist on the faculty of the University of Illinois at the time the research was done. "The nuclear changes and the morphology of the cells made it possible in most instances to tell the malignant ones from the benign ones. Identifying the malignant tumor cells made a difference in therapy." It became obvious that the next step was to use an anti-cancer chemical to kill the cancerous cells. "That was Dr. Cole's department," Dr. McGrew said.

The next year, Cole was made president of the American College of Surgeons. Founded in 1913 by a group of surgeons led by Dr. Franklin Martin, a charismatic, egotistical and controversial gynecologist and editor of a surgical journal that he started in 1905—*Surgery, Gynecology & Obstetrics*—the American College of Surgeons was dedicated to improving the standards of surgery in the United States and Canada. Cole had joined in 1929 while he was still at Washington University School of Medicine and had served on a number of important committees. In 1949 he was elected treasurer, an office he held until 1954, and from 1950 to 1951, Cole spent a year as first vice-president.

Shortly after Cole was named president-elect in 1954, Dr. Donald Balfour, who was chief of surgery at the Mayo Clinic in Rochester, Minnesota, and himself a former president of the College, wrote his congratulations:

"My dear Warren, I can't tell you how delighted I was to learn that you had been made president of the College. At this particular period in its growth, with so many important problems confronting it, your particular experience in teaching, research and activity in various organizations, your understanding of the problems of the rank and file of surgeons throughout the country and above all your judicial viewpoint will be a valuable asset. The esteem and confidence in which you are held throughout the profession and the continuity of splendid contributions which come from you and your department I know will give the College a great prestige."

Cole's mentor, Evarts Graham, was president of the College from 1940 to 1941 and served on the board of regents from 1940 to 1954, the last three years as chairman of the board. In the 1930s, Graham had fought to elevate the standards of surgery by spearheading the formation of the American Board of Surgery, an independent group that certifies the qualifications of general surgeons. At the same time, he was instrumental in raising the standards for admittance into the American College of Surgeons; now members of the College, or fellows as they are called, are required to be board-certified.

In the 1920s, the College of Surgeons initiated a hospital standardization program to upgrade the quality of care in the nation's hospitals. The program evolved into a separate organization in the 1950s, which is now known as the Joint Commission on the Accreditation of Healthcare Organizations. As did Graham early in his career, the College vehemently fought the practice of fee-splitting among surgeons and referring physicians.

Over the years, the College has had its share of detractors, some of whom scoff at its imitation of the Royal College of Surgeons of England and call it pretentious. Others consider it a stuffy and elitist "old boys' club" designed to enhance the financial status of its members. Krebiozen's promoter, Andrew Ivy, was a member of a society formed to mock the powerful American College of Surgeons, particularly its concern over unethical splitting of fees. The group was known by its Latin name, the Collegium Caninum Americanum, which translates to the American College of Dog Surgeons. The dog surgeons solemnly vowed never to "split fleas."

Nevertheless, by the time Dr. Cole became president in 1955, the American College of Surgeons was made up of the cream of the crop of American surgery, and its members influenced every aspect of the care of the surgical patient. He used his presidential address—given before about 1,000 surgeons, bedecked in royal-looking robes, who were about to become fellows of the College on November 4—to promote the idea of routine examinations for early detection of cancer. At the time, not all doctors agreed with that thought.

"Of recent years there is much discussion about the advisability of routine prophylactic examinations for cancer and other serious diseases in people who are supposedly asymptomatic," Dr. Cole said to the assembled surgeons. "Some physicians are opposed to them. Here again, I wish to say I favor the idea because we already know a certain percentage (one to two percent) of this group of people without symptoms, going to physicians, actually have a cancer. Moreover, numerous other unsuspected lesions or diseases are found (as high as 20 percent in certain reports).

"Again, I want to emphasize that we can cure most cancers if they are found early enough. We can also say that cancers are so far advanced by the time they produce significant symptoms that when patients are treated under these circumstances, the five-year survival rate is very disappointing. Accordingly, without entering the controversy as to how often routine examinations should be made, I am making this plea to respect your lay friends' request to examine them for cancer and other diseases. This examination will serve two purposes: It will ease the individual's mind and may reveal a disease which can be treated effectively in its early stages."

Cole's research in the early 1950s showed that tumor cells were not only shed at the site of operation but also went into the bloodstream of the patient, a fact that had enormous implications for the spread of cancer from one area of the body to another. Cole was not the first to find loose cancer cells around the operative site in cancer patients, but he was the first to conclude that something could and should be done to destroy them. "The medical profession has been aware of the implantation of cancer cells at the time of operation for many decades but has not fully appreciated this danger," he wrote in an editorial for the *American Surgeon* in 1959. "It was perhaps emphasized dramatically for the first time by a British surgeon named Ryall, who reported 26 instances in 1908."

In the same editorial, Cole went on to discuss the importance of cancer cells in the blood. "The demonstration of cancer cells in the peripheral blood of many patients with 'curable' cancer has led us to conclude that a great number of these dislodged cells do not survive, largely because of the host's resistance, which in the later stage of the tumor's growth decreases so much that the tumor metastasizes [spreads] widely. However, we cannot be entirely oblivious of their presence since the mechanism of death in most tumors is by vascular spread. Accordingly, the presence of cancer cells in the blood stream can certainly be considered a very unfavorable sign, and often a fatal one. It will require time to determine their true significance."

Cole hypothesized that the stress of the operation itself decreased the patient's resistance to cancer cells shed during surgery. In a separate paper published in the *American Surgeon* in 1959, he wrote of an incident that led to this conclusion. "Years ago the senior author [Cole] did a radical mastectomy on a patient with carcinoma of the breast and noted a very rapid metastatic spread of the disease thereafter. The tumor had been present for about 9 months. At operation, nodes were attached to the axillary vessels and required considerable dissection for removal. In retrospect it was rather obvious that a cure could not be expected. Within 6 weeks the patient was complaining of pain in the pelvis and back. X-rays taken a few days later revealed metastases in the lungs and pelvic bones. The patient died 6 weeks later, with extensive metastases. It actually appeared that the operation activated the tumor and made it much more invasive. Almost all surgeons have seen examples of rapid dissemination of cancer following operation, suggesting that the operation may have been a factor in the increased growth."

Nonetheless, he urged cancer surgeons not to give up on surgery in favor of alternative treatments. "The fact that operative and chemical trauma in animals appears to decrease the resistance of the animal to cancer cells, and the fact that, occasionally, cancer spreads rapidly and wildly after operation does not deter us in our conclusion that surgical treatment of cancer is the best therapeutic mechanism available. We already know what surgery will do for cancer. For example, the 5-year survival rate following resection for carcinoma of the breast, colon, rectum, and many other tumors is as high as 50 percent."

Rather, Cole's approach was to look for a chemical that might destroy the loosened cancer cells at the time of operation to prevent spread of the disease. He first investigated the effects of nitrogen mustard, and the results of his experiments would change the techniques used in cancer operations forevermore.

CHAPTER 15

⁊❧

A New Approach to Cancer Surgery

I f medical science ever finds a cure for cancer, it will probably result from the cumulative work of generations of research scientists who have labored quietly in experimental laboratories around the world. These are the people who advance our understanding of how the disease process works and how to prolong the lives of those afflicted with cancers of all sorts. Warren Cole was one of those scientists.

It might be useful to draw a comparison between Andrew Ivy and Warren Cole and their work on cancer. Both were respected researchers at the College of Medicine of the University of Illinois in the early 1950s when cancer was recognized as the number two health threat in the nation and increasing amounts of money and research were directed to its cure. But for his own inscrutable reasons, Ivy chose to go the route of the showman and ballyhoo Krebiozen to the world as a magic bullet against cancer. He jumped past the step of publishing research on the drug in respected medical journals and tried Krebiozen on cancer patients long before its biological makeup was known.

Cole, on the other hand, followed the route of sound scientific inquiry in his investigations of how cancer spreads during operations, and that made all the difference. He shunned the limelight, yet it eventually was focused on him because he made some significant and lasting discoveries. Cole was a quiet, intelligent, shy man with a quick mind and the ability to draw far-reaching conclusions from his research. He was able to tie discrete pieces of the cancer puzzle together and come up with an effective measure to help prevent the disease from spreading. When the long-awaited cure for cancer comes, it will come from the work of someone like Warren Cole, not the loud and proud Andrew Ivy.

Once Cole had published his first batch of research papers showing that cancer cells are dislodged from a tumor at the time of operation and spread to areas around the operative site as well as through the bloodstream to other parts of the patient's body, he began experiments in rats to determine if a chemical agent could be used to kill the loose cancer cells. In a paper read to the American Surgical Association in 1957, Cole explained the rationale behind his research: "Improvement in the five-year survival rate of the surgical treatment of cancer during the past ten or 15 years has been made primarily by increasing the extent of the operation. However, there is no hope that further improvement can be expected from this phase of the operation, because we are now approaching anatomic limits in respect to the amount of tissue that can be removed.

"It is natural, therefore, that we should turn our attention to the relatively recent discovery of anticancer agents. It is well known that many chemical agents will prevent the growth of cancer cells *in vitro*; some agents are effective against malignant tumors in experimental animals. However, there is no known agent which is effective in eliminating established cancer in human beings.

"Based upon animal experiments previously reported, and the knowledge that cancer cells may be disseminated by operation, we have proposed that these two methods be combined in a prophylactic or adjuvant way. The hope for success of this combined method lies in the supposition that cancer cells might be very vulnerable to the action of anticancer agents if they are given on the day of the operation, before these 'loose' cells developed a blood supply."

The animal experiments that Cole referred to were his own studies in rats, which he and his colleagues published in the August 1956 issue of the journal *Surgery*. Cole's earlier studies had proved that cancer cells lack cohesion and tend to shed, a characteristic first described by the 19th century pathologist Rudolf Virchow. Cells easily detach from a tumor and move spontaneously into blood and lymph vessels where they spread to other tissues and organs. Cole concluded that it would be easier to destroy these cells with chemicals while the cells are loose and floating, before they have a chance to reattach themselves.

In the *Surgery* article, he described how he conducted his animal experiments. "In an experimental attempt to combat venous spread of tumors of the intestinal tract, it appeared logical to use a tumor which grew well in the animal's liver, because the liver is the important site of metastases from such lesions as colon, rectum, stomach and so forth. We decided to use the Walker carcinosarcoma 256, because it was a rat tumor which grew readily in the liver when cells were injected into the portal vein, and would kill rapidly. We made a suspension of cells according to methods described by Breedis and associates and injected a suspension of 110,000 to 150,000 cells into the portal vein of control rats, and rats to be treated. We injected as many control animals as rats to be treated, and made sure that the dose was the same in the two groups of animals. We would like to emphasize that we lost a great number of animals (15 to 30 percent) from hemorrhage and other causes during the 24-hour period following injection, thus accounting for the different number of animals in the control and treated groups. We observed the animals and compared the percentage of 'takes' in the controls with those in the treated series. We are making no claim for originality in this type of experiment, but as far as we know no one has applied this principle to treatment of human cancer."

Cole and his colleagues first tried the chemical azaserine, but it had no anticancer effect in the rats. Then they used nitrogen mustard—0.25 mg. per kilogram of body weight—and found that the injected cancer cells took, or successfully attached themselves in the new host, in 97 percent of the control animals but in only 19 percent of the animals treated with nitrogen mustard. When they increased the dose to 0.5 mg. of nitrogen mustard per kilogram of body weight, the percentage of takes was 69 percent in the control animals and roughly 9 percent in the treated animals.

"It is already known that nitrogen mustard is toxic to the liver," the researchers wrote. "Yet in the treatment of advanced cancer, nitrogen mustard has been given into the peritoneal and thoracic cavities of great numbers of patients with advanced cancer without significant toxic effects." However, the animal studies showed they had to be extremely careful about when and how much nitrogen mustard they administered. "Accordingly, we realized that the margin of safety in nitrogen mustard therapy is not great. ...Nevertheless, the relative safety reported in the treatment of advanced cancer gave us assurance that the drug might be given with reasonable safety on the day of operation."

In March 1956, armed with the results of successful studies in animals, Cole and his research team began experiments on human cancer patients. They injected nitrogen mustard into patients undergoing operations for cancer of the breast, lung, colon, rectum or stomach on the day of operation and for three days afterward. "We have already learned that the toxicity of nitrogen mustard is much more significant in the freshly operated patient than in other patients, and logically so, because the patient operated on for a cancer has sustained a rather severe load," they wrote for *Surgery* in August 1956 (the other authors were Ernesto P. Cruz, M.D., and Gerald O. McDonald, M.D.).

In a follow-up study published in the *Annals of Surgery* in 1957, Cole and colleagues (Francisco Morales, M.D., Millar Bell, M.B., and Gerald O. McDonald, M.D.) reported: "When we began the adjuvant treatment of human cancer with nitrogen mustard at the time of operation, we were immediately confronted with the question as to whether it would be preferable to give the anticancer agent all at one time on the day of operation, or in divided doses to afford safety, and likewise expose the tumor to an anticancer agent at different stages of cell mitoses." So they conducted a series of animal experiments to show what happened when nitrogen mustard was given at various times before and after cancer cells were injected into rats. As a result, they settled on four daily doses beginning on the day of operation.

"Utilizing a total dosage level of 0.4 mgm. per kilogram body weight, we established a treatment protocol excluding all patients 70 years old or older. At the completion of surgery, one-fourth the total dose (0.1 mgm. per kilogram of body weight) was administered. Those patients with gastrointestinal tract malignancies receive this first dose directly into the peritoneal cavity at the completion of surgery, the drug first being diluted in 400 ml. physiologic saline. Patients with carcinoma of the breast receive that first dose intravenously at the completion of surgery. The subsequent doses are administered to both groups intravenously on the first three postoperative days. Any one day's dose was limited to a maximum of 7.5 mgm. to eliminate overdosage in fat people."

They later changed the protocol so that half the total was administered at the time of operation because the effects of nitrogen mustard diminish as time elapses after operation, and experience taught them it was safe to increase the dose.

The studies were so promising that the National Cancer Institute, through its National Cancer Chemotherapy Center, organized a clinical trial of Cole's cancer therapy in clinics throughout the country. The treatment had its greatest benefit in patients operated on for cancer of the breast. Cole also continued his studies, and by the end of 1959 was able to report: "Up to April 1959, we have treated 74 patients with cancer of the breast by the prophylactic or adjuvant method; half were controls. There have been 12 recurrences and 7 deaths from cancer in the control patients, and 5 recurrences and 1 death from cancer in the treated patients. This reveals a very favorable trend, but the series is too small to be statistically significant. Accordingly, we consider the procedure entirely experimental and do not yet advise it for routine use. If this method of therapy stands the test of time, we would not expect one chemical to be effective for all tumors."

In fact, the therapy did stand the test of time, and adjuvant chemotherapy, a term used to describe the use of anticancer chemicals in combination with surgery to fight the spread of cancer, is routinely used all over the world. In the late 1950s, some 30,000 to 40,000 chemicals were tested every year to determine their effectiveness against various types of cancer. As Dr. Cole predicted in his early research, different tumors respond to different chemicals and there proved to be no single agent that was effective against all cancers.

When Cole was doing his research in the 1950s, surgery and radiation therapy were the two measures that could effectively stop cancer growth. Paul Ehrlich (1854-1915) is generally recognized as the father of chemotherapy, but it was not until 1941 when Charles Huggins began to use estrogens in the treatment of prostate cancer that the modern era of cancer therapy with chemicals and hormones began. Thanks to Dr. Cole's early work in adjuvant chemotherapy and the work of other pioneers in cancer chemotherapy, as well as the follow-up research conducted by the National Cancer Institute, chemotherapy is now widely used alone or in combination with surgery and radiation in the fight against cancer. Today, modern medicine recognizes that cancer is not a single disease but a huge number of different diseases that require a variety of therapeutic approaches.

Cole became a recognized expert in adjuvant chemotherapy, and in 1970 he published a medical textbook on the use of chemotherapy, called *Chemotherapy of Cancer*.

"Of all Dr. Cole's contributions," said Dr. LaSalle D. Leffall, Jr., chairman of the department of surgery at Howard University College of Medicine in Washington, D.C., and a former president of the American Cancer Society, in an interview in 1990, "his work on circulating cancer cells and the clinical implications of that is the most important. At that time, it was a real contribution."

In recognition of his contributions to cancer research, the American Cancer Society elected Dr. Cole president in 1959 for a one-year term. The American Cancer Society evolved from the American Society for the Control of Cancer, an organization formed by a small group of physicians in 1913 for the purpose of spreading information about the treatment and prevention of cancer in language that the public could understand. In 1945, Mary Lasker, the wife of a wealthy industrialist, spearheaded an effort to raise funds for the ASCC that would go toward research into the causes of cancer. She and her cohorts raised $10 million in 1946, and the Board of

Directors changed the name of the organization to the American Cancer Society. In 1959, the society had two million members and it was recognized as one of the world's most effective forces working to halt cancer.

"In the past decade," Dr. Cole said in his presidential address at the society's annual meeting on October 26, 1960, "the number of compounds screened in the search for a possible chemical treatment has reached into the hundreds of thousands. From this wide spectrum, perhaps a score have been found which can be found useful in human cancer. Strangely enough, one of the first, amethopterin, which was extensively used in treating leukemia for some years, now appears to be the first compound truly effective against a solid tumor. Known by another trade name of methotrexate, this substance has apparently resulted in complete regression of a number of cases of choriocarcinoma, a rare form of cancer usually occurring in connection with childbirth.

"The random search for chemicals has now given way to a more precise method of building molecules with certain qualities designed to attack the cellular growth processes through their enzyme pathways. Such an approach seems to be zeroing in on the target with much greater promise. As an example, we might mention 5-FU (5-fluorouracil), which was developed by one of your society's so-called lifetime grantees, Charles Heidelberger of the University of Wisconsin, a man who is dedicating his entire career to cancer research. The important factor in this work is that it was an entirely new type of chemical, with a new means of attacking the cancer cell."

Cole went on to say, "New chemicals are appearing now almost on an assembly line basis. Although no one drug actually has resulted in a five-year cure of human cancer, many are useful, particularly in the leukemias, extending by months and even years the lives of many of those who previously died within a few short weeks."

By 1960, medical science was well aware that the environment plays a significant role in the development of cancer. Cigarette smoking was an obvious example. After World War II, cigarette consumption skyrocketed, and so did the incidence of lung cancer. In his speech to the cancer society, Dr.

Cole railed against smoking in his flat Midwestern style. "Epidemiological studies have clearly proved that certain substances could cause cancer—how they cause it we still don't know—but the case against such carcinogens as occur in cigarette smoke is so strong that it seems certain now that some 20,000 lives a year are the cost the American public pays for this luxury.

"Those who would take comfort from the belief that scientists are not in agreement as to how cigarette tars and viruses might both be causes of neoplasms are being misled, for cancer appears to be a disease with multiple causes. Many virologists, firm in their theory that viruses are involved in human cancer, are nonetheless convinced that regular cigarette smokers are some ten times more likely to get lung cancer than nonsmokers. Actually, there is no conflict between the two viewpoints. If it is demonstrated that viruses are a causative agent in lung cancer, the carcinogens in cigarette smoke will certainly be found to act in concert with them. The fact remains that today we have no means of eliminating the virus, even if it does exist, but there is a way of removing the cigarette tar—remove the cigarette from your mouth."

At the same time that he was doing research on adjuvant chemotherapy, Dr. Cole was looking into another aspect of cancer that had long confounded clinicians—-the spontaneous regression of cancer. Simply put, spontaneous regression means that the cancer disappears altogether or decreases in size either temporarily or permanently. In 1901, Sir William Osler was sufficiently convinced of the phenomenon that he published a paper describing two cases of regression among breast cancer patients. One of the patients had been given a radical mastectomy by William S. Halsted in October 1897. Later the cancer spread to another part of the body but that tumor mass disappeared over the course of two years.

With a grant from the American Cancer Society and the Illinois Federated Women's Clubs, Cole and Dr. Tilden Everson, clinical professor of surgery in Cole's department at the University of Illinois, undertook a study of spontaneous regression as reported in medical literature around the world since 1900. They presented a preliminary report of their findings to a meeting of the American Surgical Association on

April 11, 1956.

In a guest editorial published in the *Journal of the American Medical Association* on April 11, 1959—ironically along with a staff-written editorial urging that the Krebiozen Research Foundation cooperate with the National Cancer Institute in a scientific evaluation of Krebiozen—Cole and Everson wrote:

"For decades the reported disappearance of malignant tumors, without significant therapy to explain it, has intrigued the profession, and has given rise to controversy as to whether or not the phenomenon actually exists. Spontaneous regression of cancer may be defined as the partial or complete disappearance of a malignant tumor in the absence of all treatment or in the presence of therapy which is considered inadequate to exert a significant influence on the growth of neoplastic disease. Indeed, spontaneous regression is a somewhat inaccurate term for this phenomenon because any change in the growth pattern of malignant tissue must have a biological explanation.

"Efforts to find an explanation of this phenomenon have been thwarted by the fact that, fortunately, only a small fraction of patients with malignant disease go untreated. Thus, spontaneous regression of cancer has been mainly reported in patients in whom the cancer was beyond the scope of cure by the accepted techniques of surgery and/or radiation."

In addition to studying reports in medical journals, they also solicited unpublished reports of spontaneous regression from medical and surgical colleagues. By the time Cole and Everson published a book on the subject in 1966, they had collected a total of 176 cases that they felt were adequately documented to prove the existence of spontaneous regression of cancer. Previous investigators had estimated that cancers regress spontaneously in as few as one in 100,000 cancer patients, although it is impossible to determine that number accurately.

In a 1974 interview with the editor of *CA*, a medical journal devoted to cancer, Dr. Cole remarked, "I am convinced that there is no single explanation but rather many causes. After careful analysis of our 176 patients, we were able to group all the incidents or factors that could be related to spontaneous regression of cancer into seven categories. They include hormones, drugs, removal of a carcinogen, immune reaction, irradiation, operative trauma, fever and/or infection. Although one or all of these might exert a role in the spontaneous regression of cancer, I have no proof."

Farther on in the interview, he said that he found only 15 patients in whom regression could be attributed to the fact that they were removed from exposure to an environmental carcinogen. Cole traced most of the regressions to a direct or indirect immune response inside the patients. "In fact," he said, "I believe that increased immunologic resistance, either temporary or permanent, is the most significant explanation for most spontaneous regressions of cancer."

When the editor asked how many of the 176 cases could be attributed to the patients' natural immune system, Cole responded, "The question should really be answered in two parts. First, we documented only 14 cases of spontaneous regression that were linked to possible immunologic factors. The most dramatic examples occurred in three patients with malignant melanomas. In one patient, the tumor regressed after a blood transfusion from a patient who previously had a spontaneous regression of melanoma; in another, regression followed a transfusion from a patient who had a 10-year cure after radical excision of a melanoma; and in a third patient, regression followed three transfusions from the blood bank, the last of which was blood group A, Rh-negative.

"In addition to these few examples, however, I believe that many other cases of spontaneous regression associated with operative trauma, irradiation and infection are more adequately explained by an immunologic mechanism."

In the *JAMA* editorial, Cole and Everson concluded that their research might offer some hope to incurable cancer patients. "The remote possibility of spontaneous regression of cancer may be of some psychotherapeutic value in offering hope to patients and relatives of patients with 'incurable' cancer. Often, indeed, the mere thought that regression might possibly take place changes their attitude from that of complete despair to that of hopeful toleration. The profession should use knowledge of this phenomenon, rare as it is, in an endeavor to comfort the patient and his relatives in the trying days of terminal cancer. With proper precaution the physician can do this without being guilty of offering false hopes."

It was his work in cancer research that led Cole to national and international acclaim recognizing his lasting contributions to medical care. Cholecystography gave him fame, but his cancer studies showed that his fame was not fleeting nor his brilliance short-lived.

CHAPTER 16

ઢ

ADVANCING EDUCATION
IN SURGERY

T hink what you will about Andrew Ivy, the man was an outstanding fundraiser. Through his efforts, the University of Illinois professional colleges in Chicago went on a building spree in the early 1950s in response to increased enrollments following World War II, and Warren Cole finally got the expanded research hospital he had wanted since 1936 when he first went to Illinois.

New student housing went up to accommodate medical school classes of 150 or more. By 1953, the addition to the research hospital was completed and another general hospital opened in the medical center complex—the West Side Veterans Administration Hospital, which gave the medical school a new resource for teaching and research. The university also began to beef up its full-time clinical staff to join Cole and Dr. Henry Poncher, another full-time department head who was hired during the war.

In 1950, Dr. Harry Dowling was named full-time head of the department of preventive medicine, and the next year he became head of the department of medicine. Writing for the centennial issue of the Illini *Scope*, Dowling recalled the professional atmosphere at Illinois when he arrived to interview for his appointment. "Henry Poncher was chairing the committee to select a head of the newly created Department of

Preventive Medicine. Energetic and bursting with ideas, he had built an active, socially-oriented Department of Pediatrics containing six young, vigorous, full-time faculty members, among them Julius Richmond, later to become Surgeon General of the U.S. Public Health Service.

"The other full-time clinicians in the medical college were Warren Cole, head of the Department of Surgery, who was working 70 hours a week or more to keep his hospital service up to standards; and Carroll Birch and Robert Kark, in the Department of Medicine. Poncher and Dean John Youmans assured me that both faculty and administration were committed to developing a core group of full-time faculty in each of the larger departments."

But while Andrew Ivy helped foster the growth of the professional colleges at Illinois in the early 1950s, he also brought a loss of prestige to the university and a black eye to the College of Medicine's research and teaching image as a result of his defense of Krebiozen. After the university's president George Stoddard banned further clinical research on Krebiozen at Illinois in 1952 and the board of trustees fired Stoddard in 1953, the College of Medicine lost a stream of reputable faculty members and department heads and found it difficult to entice suitable replacements to the positions.

Despite the defections, however, Warren Cole stayed and continued to build his department's reputation. He had fought to eliminate the didactic teaching tradition that remained at Illinois through the 1940s but advocated retaining some form of formal instruction. "In the late '40s our medical school, as did all others, began consideration of abolishment of all didactic teaching," he wrote for the *Scope* in 1981. "I favored the plan, but I differed from many in that I had a firm belief that there must be a substitute for the didactic plan, so that we could be sure the student would have the factual data about a disease so he could make a diagnosis and develop a plan of therapy.

"Some clinicians had the idea our faculty could supply that factual data as we walked around the wards with the students. It was obvious to me that there are not enough hours of ward walks to supply the didactic needs.

"I contend that relying on the student to obtain a valid

picture of the symptoms and signs about a disease from one patient (or two or three) is invalid reasoning because no two examples of a disease are alike. Textbooks are designed to present these irregularities of disease. It takes much less time for a student to read about the characteristics of a disease than it does to talk about them. To expect the physician to know medicine without a knowledge of symptoms and signs is similar to expecting an engineer to carry on his practical duties without a basic knowledge of mathematics.

"The hope of many of our faculty was that the student would voluntarily do the necessary reading. In my experience, the top third of the class will do that, but the rest will fail to a variable degree. We made up this deficiency by formation of a very informed course during the surgical quarter discussing important subjects, but with reading assignments. No examination was held, although one was held at the end of the junior year."

In his annual report to the dean of the College of Medicine, dated June 21, 1950, Dr. Cole described the surgical training available to students at the time: "In the sophomore year, we have a seminar class consisting of 12 hours during the last quarter, in which certain subjects, such as surgical bacteriology, infections, wounds, etc., are discussed. In addition to this, we have an equal number of hours for surgical physical diagnosis.

"The juniors are assigned to clerkships on the ward for one quarter. Thirty are assigned to Illinois Research Hospital, 16 to Presbyterian and nine to Cook County Hospital. In general, I believe that we have a very good clerkship here at Illinois Research Hospital and at Presbyterian, but I am by no means happy about the clerkship at Cook County Hospital, largely because of our inability to have students scrub in the operating room with the surgical team. At all three hospitals, the students spend the greater part of their time on the ward, but are assembled once or twice a day for formal discussion of patients.

"During the senior year, the students have dispensary [outpatient clinic] work as a major part of their assignment. Twelve students are sent to St. Luke's Hospital for six weeks and 12 to the Orthopedic Institute for six weeks. For the remaining six weeks, each of these two groups is assigned to the various surgical dispensaries. Six senior students are sent to Presbyterian Hospital. They stay over there the entire quarter and get their dispensary work there."

Inspired by a system of medical instruction used in Paris, Vienna and Dublin, the clinical clerkship is a time-honored method of teaching medicine that was first introduced in the United States in 1857 at the New Orleans School of Medicine. Under the plan, students are assigned individual patients to study during their entire hospital stays, from admission to discharge. Medical students take detailed histories of the patients, perform complete physical exams and discuss their findings with the professor or resident, who uses the patient as a teaching example and makes recommendations for management. In the 1890s, Johns Hopkins established the clerkship as a permanent fixture of medical education.

With the rise of university-affiliated medical schools and research hospitals, clerkships became universally available, although few schools allowed clinical clerks a great deal of responsibility. At some schools, the hospital rotation came in the junior year, while seniors worked in the clinics; in other schools, the reverse was true. In fact, Dr. Cole changed Illinois' clerkship year from the senior year to the junior year in 1948. Despite its widespread appeal, medical educators debate the fine line between education and cheap labor that the clerkship often crosses.

In his 1950 annual report, Cole also described postgraduate training in his department of surgery: "Our program is devoted almost entirely to training of research fellows, residents and interns. We have no routine postgraduate courses. Each research fellow is expected to attend our surgical conferences, including particularly the research seminar on Saturday mornings, surgical pathology on Thursday afternoon and the journal club on Monday afternoon. In addition, the men registered in the graduate school must attend two or three seminars per week in any of the other departments. In addition, they are expected to attend ward rounds conducted by the head of the department four afternoons per week for about an hour and half each day. These ward rounds are designed specifically for scientific teaching."

Sir Geoffrey Slaney, who was head of the department of surgery at Queen Elizabeth Hospital, Birmingham University, in Birmingham, England, from 1971 to 1986, and a former president of the Royal College of Surgeons of England (1982-86), studied under Dr. Cole as a research fellow in 1956. "Following the war, surgical research was in its infancy," Sir Geoffrey said in an interview in 1990, "and there was a growing recognition of its import in most of the youngsters of my age group. In the early 1950s, a relatively small number of young English surgeons were interested in going to the States to study principally research methods rather than clinical attachments, although we were very keen to get a handle on any clinical experience we could find." His chief of surgery knew Dr. Cole and arranged for Sir Geoffrey to spend a year under Cole's wing.

"It was the time in Dr. Cole's program when the recognition of the dissemination of cancer by circulating cancer cells was just coming on stream," Sir Geoffrey recalled. "The thing that impressed me first about him was that he was an excellent clinical surgeon. I had come from a background where clinical surgery was very highly rated. But the thing that came to amaze me was his depth of interest in research and his knowledge of research. At the time, he had something like 12 young surgeons from all over the world in his laboratory, including three or four Americans, all actively engaged in pursuing important avenues of research.

"I found him a very impressive teacher. Every Saturday morning he would hold a meeting, which I think started about 10, and all the chaps in the lab had to be there. We sat around a table with Dr. Cole at the head. We all had to give a report of what we had done that week, what snags we were running into, what the good bits were and all the rest of it. He would listen to it all and say something like, 'That's very interesting, but of course if you do it that way, I would predict'—that was one of his favorite aphorisms—'I would predict you are going to have trouble. I'm sure if you go back and look in the *Annals* about 1947, you'll find a similar problem.' Here were these dozen young chaps beavering away, really up with the literature and everything that was going on, and I never heard him at a loss, not once, to make a constructive comment. I learned so much from him."

Everybody in postgraduate study, whether in the research program or the clinical program, was expected to be present at ward rounds, Sir Geoffrey said. "Whenever he made rounds, he had his research fellows with him, and they took part in the clinical decisions. So although you were doing a lab program, you got this tie-in to what the clinical activity of the department was."

Dr. Cole felt his Saturday meetings with residents, interns and research fellows were so sacrosanct that if, for example, he had a Friday night speech on the West Coast, he would try to catch an overnight plane back to Chicago to keep from missing the Saturday seminar. "The example he set was so impressive," Sir Geoffrey said. "Ward rounds would go on until 4:00 on Saturday afternoon. That was unknown in the U.K. We would have the research meeting on Saturday morning until at least noon and then the rounds would start at about 1:00. We would just about have time for a hamburger and had to go back."

Dr. Cole stood about 5'9" and weighed a slight 145 pounds, yet many of his students considered him intimidating. "He had a reserve, and at first, I think, everybody found him formidable, but I found him very easy to talk to," said Sir Geoffrey. "I know that many of my contemporaries in the residency program were scared and I could never quite fathom that. I began to realize later on that it was a facet of the residency program—you had to watch your Ps and Qs. He had absolute authority to hire and fire. Yet his ex-residents hold him not only with regard but with quite a measure of affection. It was understood that if you were working for Warren Cole, you were expected to lay it on the line and do your best."

The 1950s saw the rapid development of specialization in surgery, a process that began in the United States with ophthalmology in the early 1800s. The disciplines of orthopedic surgery and ear, nose, and throat surgery emerged in the mid-1800s, followed by urology and obstetrics in the late 1800s. Harvey Cushing pioneered the field of brain surgery after the turn of the century, and thoracic surgery emerged before World War I. Plastic surgery came into its own between the wars, and colon and rectal surgery was formally recognized as a surgical discipline in 1949. But in the next 30 years, medical knowledge exploded and so did specialization. By the mid-1980s, the *Directory of Medical Specialists*, published by the American Medical Association, listed 81 medical specialties, 22 of them related to surgery.

However, in terms of surgical education and research, general surgery has remained the unifying discipline that all other specialties of surgery depend upon. Training in general surgery immediately following medical school has provided the basis for specialization later on in residency training, and the in-depth research conducted in broad areas of surgery since World War II has led to the very definition of the surgical specialties.

Thus in the 1950s, Dr. Cole was faced with the dilemma of providing students with both basic training in general surgery and the opportunity to study the various surgical specialties. Medical educators debated the best method of meeting this dilemma. In his retirement years, Cole wrote an essay on the subject that describes his approach to teaching general surgery.

"Should there be an ideal residency program used by all departments of surgery?" he asked. "The answer to this is no, and decisively so. The reason is that there are so many different types of training programs available that we could not include all the good aspects of them in one program. Furthermore, we already know that the candidate himself or herself does not want to be confined to certain patterns in his training program. So often circumstances change, and the candidate wants to substitute a certain program in his curriculum for one of the so-called standard features.

"We must admit that following the advice and limitations set by the American Board of Surgery, a large variation of programs is possible, and justifiably so. I am in favor of accepting variations, except that unless care is exercised, too many electives are sometimes allowed and certain of the minor specialties may be omitted completely from the candidate's curriculum. I think it is better to make sure that no important specialties are omitted and that the 'attractive' electives are included as graduate studies to be taken up later."

Cole pointed to his mentor Evarts Graham as an example of someone who did not have a formal residency in surgery but rather spent seven years in research in the basic sciences and emerged as a gifted surgical scientist. Because of his own year in the research lab working on cholecystography, Cole felt strongly that a year of pure research was of great value to the surgical trainee. In his presidential address to the American College of Surgeons in 1955, he said:

"Comparison of methods of teaching surgery a few decades ago and at the present time reveals a rather sharp contrast, obviously for the better. Without going into details, let me remind you that three or four decades ago teaching of surgery was carried out primarily by the apprenticeship method, whereas at the present time the major teaching program is carried out in a hospital in a residency. We have learned comparatively recently that a year in research is of tremendous advantage to the surgeon in his practice. It teaches the young surgeon a lot of fundamental facts about physiology and numerous other basic sciences; likewise, it encourages him to apply scientific methods in solving clinical problems, and should also instill a scientific curiosity of a lasting type in the mind and soul of the surgeon."

Sir Geoffrey Slaney recalled his year with Warren Cole as a turning point in his surgical career. "He put me to work with two of Ormand Julian's research fellows who were trying to develop the first heart-lung machine down at the R & E [Illinois' Research and Educational Hospitals]. John Kirklin was beavering away at the Mayo on the same thing. We used to spend days with this curious sort of scaffolding frame with bags hanging off it and bubbling oxygen. All terribly crude. But that meant that I started going to Ormand Julian's operating sessions. Now I wasn't interested in cardiac surgery because that had become a separate specialty, but vascular surgery was just starting to be developed for peripheral vessels. I saw Ormand do some of the early aortic prosthetic replacements, and that's where I began to get an increasing feeling that this would be an interesting field to develop back home. So it was through my work with Warren Cole as a general surgeon that I came back with this interest in vascular surgery."

The length of surgical residency programs varies according to the specialty and the final goal of the resident. "Some residencies are 10 or 12 years long," Dr. Cole wrote in his retirement years. "In general, the professor is training these men to be heads of departments. Actually Dr. Halsted of Johns Hopkins originated this long residency. Many residency programs add two or three years of training in non-clinical sciences so that the resident obtains a PhD as well. Such residencies must be six or seven years long. They are particularly useful for those going into academic surgery because PhD training is so helpful in research.

"Three of my last ten residents came to me in the middle of their residency asking for advice about continued education. Each had had a year in the surgical laboratory in addition to three years of clinical work on the wards. I actually believe that a year in the laboratory is valuable for any young surgeon, even though he plans to go into clinical and not academic surgery.

"Each of the three residents was really inquiring about academic life since all were anxious to obtain a position in a medical school doing research as well as working on the wards and teaching. Each had done some research work (mostly in cancer) and liked it and wanted to continue in research. I told each of them I thought their choice was appropriate and wise, but that if they were going to continue doing research throughout their lives, they would have to get PhD-type training, including much work in immunology. All accepted my advice and obtained a PhD or its equivalent. At that time (the late 1950s and early 1960s), there was a demand for young surgeons with training of that type, so they readily obtained positions in my department or elsewhere.

"Not much has been said or written about the needs of a young surgeon training for an academic career versus one training for a clinical career. By an academic career, I mean a career as a medical school faculty member, where the surgeon is expected to do part-time research, write articles appropriate to his specialty, teach medical students and spend some time in the operating room.

"In my opinion, the academic surgeon should be as highly educated as possible. He can improve his education considerably by taking many science courses as electives throughout his educational career. This will also improve his competitive value when candidates are being considered for promotions. The extra science courses—genetics, advanced immunology, cellular immunology, immunological research, advanced biochemistry, advanced hematology, virology, differential equations, advanced organic chemistry, biophysics, fluids and electrolytes, and computer science—will help the surgeon produce medical papers.

"The atmosphere created by various teachers in the department is very important in stimulating ideas in the minds of young surgeons. Naturally, the head of the department is important in helping to stimulate ideas for publication.

"The clinical surgeon who goes out into practice must face as much competition as the academic surgeon, but it is of a different type. Of course, the surgeon in practice must be as well educated as possible, but education is not as important as it is for the academic surgeon. More important to the clinical surgeon's armament is his personality, which is often referred to as his bed-side manner. In my opinion, advanced physiology is probably the most valuable elective course for the clinical surgeon. Advanced pathology may also be very useful."

Dr. Olga Jonasson, one of Cole's residents in the 1960s who subsequently became chief of surgery at Cook County Hospital and then the Robert M. Zollinger Professor and chairman of the department of surgery at Ohio State University, remembered how Cole influenced her training for academic life. "I had always thought I would go into academics and I assumed I would just stay on at the University of Illinois, but Dr. Cole told me that I needed to go away and do research training. It was the best advice he could ever have given. I really was not ready to enter the faculty at that time. He then helped me get a fellowship.

"I went to Walter Reed Army Institute of Research in Washington, D.C., working for an immunochemist. I was very unhappy there because I had no clinical work at all. I came back to Chicago that Thanksgiving and asked Dr. Cole to take me back at Illinois. He said, 'No, you've got to finish what you started.' So I went back and took a couple of other research fellowships. Without that research training, I never would have advanced. It was critical to my entire career.

"Dr. Cole was clearly the major influence on my life because he was such a marvelous role model," Dr. Jonasson said. "He was exactly the type of doctor that I thought I always wanted to be—knowledgeable, careful, thorough, compassionate."

When the addition to Illinois' research hospital was built in 1953, an emergency room service was planned and implemented. Dr. Cole was put in charge of the service. "Much planning went into the arrangements for the service, as we recognized that adequate facilities as well as personnel are necessary to conduct a good teaching program and, at the same time, render good service to the injured or sick patient," he told surgeons attending a meeting of the Metropolitan Chicago Chapter of the American College of Surgeons in 1955.

Cole appointed Dr. John Schneewind, who had just finished his term as senior resident in Cole's department, as chief of the emergency service, effective when the service opened on October 1, 1954. Together, Cole and Schneewind began building an effective service and writing and speaking about their experiences to their medical colleagues.

This new responsibility thrust Cole into the center of a growing issue in medical education. The incidence of accidental death and injury was increasing at an alarming rate, primarily because of the burgeoning of the American love affair with the automobile. More and more highways were built to accommodate more and more automobiles that were driven at higher and higher speeds.

At the same time, with the growth of specialization in medicine, the general practitioner was fast becoming an anachronism and people began to use hospital emergency rooms as their entry to the health-care system, whether or not their ailments constituted true emergencies. As was true with his cancer research, Cole moved into the forefront of a major national health issue at a time when attention was being focused on it. Accidental death would eventually become the nation's fourth leading killer, following heart disease, cancer and stroke, and the need for trained physicians for the emergency room was to become critical.

Cole's role in defining an emergency service and the medical training necessary for those who staff it enhanced his reputation as a guiding authority in medical education and led to an appointment that would allow him to leave a lasting mark on the training of all young doctors, not just surgeons.

CHAPTER 17

THE NEW FLEXNERS

I n his annual report for 1956-57, Dr. Cole wrote about the emergency service he set up at the University of Illinois Research and Educational Hospitals. "The emergency service began operation on October 1, 1954, in order to provide facilities for the teaching of emergency care of acutely ill and injured patients to our interns, residents and students. In view of the general increase in accident rates throughout the country due to high-speed motor cars, the teaching of trauma has become a vital part of any complete program. In addition, the emergency service forms an integral part of the plan for treating mass casualties which may occur as a result of local disasters, such as bus accidents and wind storms, or the treatment of casualties on an even larger scale in the event of a national catastrophe."

In the vein of the true scientist, Cole began to quantify and categorize the numbers and types of patients who used his emergency room. "Very few individuals appreciate the great variety of conditions which will appear in the emergency service," he and Dr. Schneewind wrote for the *American Journal of Surgery* in 1959. "When one thinks of the emergency room, a lacerated arm or gunshot wound immediately comes to mind. However, these represent only a small fraction of the emergency conditions seen in a busy emergency service. In a twelve-month period between July 1, 1957, and July 1, 1958, 15,841 patients were seen in our emergency service. However, only 18.2 percent of their conditions were traumatic."

They reported that some 27 percent of the 15,841 patients were treated by surgery, while more than 18 percent were sent to the medical service for treatment and another 18 percent were given pediatric care. The rest of the emergency-room patients required treatment from a wide variety of hospital specialists. "Accordingly," they wrote, "an emergency service involves every specialty in the hospital, and every specialty must take part in preparation of the teaching program."

In 1956, when Cole was president of the American Association for the Surgery of Trauma, he devoted his presidential address to describing what he had learned in setting up a teaching program for emergency care. "I believe the responsibility of a busy emergency unit is so great that it almost requires a full-time surgeon." Surgeons were initially in charge of emergency rooms in hospitals around the country. After the 1950s, specialists in emergency-room care began to emerge; some were trauma surgeons, some emergency-room physicians.

As the emergency service evolved at Illinois, Cole and Schneewind learned a few things the hard way about placing interns in charge of the emergency room. "In our emergency room at the Illinois Research Hospital," Cole said in his presidential address, "we have students, interns and residents in training. The intern is the physician in charge. We have learned through somewhat bitter experience that he must be put through a period of education and indoctrination for several days before he begins his duties. Otherwise, he will make numerous mistakes, some of which may be serious, before he learns the various precautions and principles in the care of the injured patient.

"The intern is told above everything else not to assume responsibility if there is the slightest doubt that his decision may be wrong. If he is not sure about the accuracy of his decision, he must call the resident in charge of the service to which the patient would be assigned. If the resident is not certain about the accuracy of his opinion, he must call the attending man on duty. Every night a trained surgeon is on call in our emergency room to accept responsibility. Some of the problems can be settled over the telephone, but many indeed will require the attending surgeon to go to the emergency room and see the patient. Needless to say, no surgeon should be assigned to night calls in an emergency service more than twice a week."

Cole urged that a method of certifying surgeons who treat trauma patients in the emergency room be established by the American Board of Surgery, which the board subsequently did. Cole's influence with the American Board of Surgery was strong; he spent a term from 1951 to 1953 as chairman of the board. He also urged that residents in all the specialties have at least some training in the emergency room.

Cole's studies of the types of patients who visited emergency rooms served to underline a fundamental shift that was taking place in medicine in the United States—the rise of specialization and the decline of the general practitioner. Fewer and fewer physicians were serving as family physicians to whom patients could go for a wide range of health problems. In 1931, 84 percent of all physicians in private practice were general practitioners and only 15 percent were specialists. By 1960, the percentage of GPs had declined to 45 percent, and by 1965, it had slid further to 37 percent, many of whom were over 65 years old. In the early 1960s, a mere 15 percent of all medical school graduates had planned to enter general practice.

In 1962, recognizing this shift and the need to reform graduate medical education to respond to it, the American Medical Association appointed a commission, called the Citizens Commission on Graduate Medical Education, to study the problem and make recommendations. The commission was designed to do for graduate medical education what Flexner had done for undergraduate medical education 50 years earlier.

While four of the 12 members of the commission were physicians, the remaining eight members represented a variety of disciplines. One was a former U.S. Supreme Court

Justice, two were university presidents, one was a professor
of sociology, two were businessmen and one was an executive with the American Association for the Advancement
of Science.

Of the four physicians, one was a past president of the
American Medical Association, another was the former dean
of Western Reserve University School of Medicine, the third
was assistant professor of medicine at Western Reserve who
acted as secretary to the commission and the fourth was Warren H. Cole, the only surgeon appointed to the commission.

Presiding as chairman was John S. Millis, president of
Western Reserve University in Cleveland. The Citizens Commission became popularly known as the Millis Commission,
and it was to have a lasting effect on the future of graduate
medical education.

In the introduction to the Millis Commission's report,
published in 1966 and titled *The Graduate Education of
Physicians*, the members of the commission observed: "Medical education and the practice for which it gives preparation
face problems quite different in kind but nearly as profound
as those which concerned Abraham Flexner half a century
ago. When Flexner wrote, medical education and practice
were suffering from the lack of a solid, scientific base. Now,
the scientific base not only exists but has grown so explosive-
ly that it has outrun much of medical practice. Then, medical
education suffered from the lack of effective standards. A
problem of today is the complexity, the fragmentation, and
the inflexibility of standards for graduate medical education.
When Flexner conducted his inquiry into medical education,
the public was little concerned. Now the public is deeply concerned."

"The American Medical Association wanted to obtain an
idea of the worthiness of graduate medical education," Dr.
Cole said of his experience on the commission, "and especially to determine what should be done about the general practitioner, who was receiving so much criticism about his medical performance.

"All specialists were given three to five years of training
in their field before they were allowed to go out into practice," Dr. Cole said. "They were also compelled to take and

pass an examination given by a board of physicians who were trained and practicing in that specialty. The examination made certain that patients would receive medical care from a physician who was highly trained in one of the various specialties.

"However, the general practitioner could go into practice the day he finished medical school, provided he passed an examination given by the state in which he was to practice. It is true, however, that he usually spent one year in an internship. In the early days, most of the internships were of the rotating type, giving training in surgery, internal medicine and obstetrics and gynecology, with a brief exposure to other specialties, such as psychiatry, dermatology and neurology.

"One can readily see that this year of training in the various specialties would be entirely inadequate to supply the knowledge the general practitioner needed to act as a diagnostician and referring agent to the proper specialist if he encountered a disease too complicated or advanced for him to take care of."

The Millis Commission's first line of attack was to recommend that a separate year of internship be abolished and the training absorbed by the residency system. The members of the commission argued that the clinical clerkship in undergraduate medical schools had taken the place of the rotating internship. "Because nearly all students now go on from an internship to a residency, the nature of the internship has changed," the commission's report stated. "The original, or rotating, form provides from 12 to 24 months of experience in medicine, surgery, pediatrics, and obstetrics-gynecology. More recently two other forms have come into use: mixed internships—which resemble rotating internships in providing training in two or three fields, but differ by requiring that from six to eight months be spent in one field; and straight internships—which are devoted entirely to single areas, such as medicine, surgery, or pediatrics." The straight internship differed little from residency training, except for the level of responsibility.

But if the internship were abolished, there remained the question of what to do about the general practitioner in light of the explosion in medical knowledge. "The commission spent nearly three years studying this problem," Dr. Cole recalled. "Toward the end, I was asked point-blank what I would recommend for the general practitioner. Should he be preserved as a specialty? I said I thought he should be preserved but must be compelled to undertake a residency program of at least three years. After detailed discussion, the commission recommended three years of residency training for the general practitioner."

The commission proposed that the old idea of the general practitioner be molded into a new specialty known as the primary physician. "There is an annoying semantic problem in talking about this kind of physician," the commission's report intoned. "What should he be called? The title general practitioner has lost its once honored status. Dr. Russell Lee suggests that we 'build a monument to him and...start now with a new concept of the personal physician.'"

"We suggest that he be called a primary physician. He should usually be primary in the first-contact sense. He will serve as the primary medical resource and counselor to an individual or a family. When a patient needs hospitalization, the services of other medical specialists, or other medical or paramedical assistance, the primary physician will see that the necessary arrangements are made, giving such responsibility to others as appropriate, and retaining his own continuing and comprehensive responsibility."

The ideal place for the primary physician to practice, the report said, is in group practice. "Practice within a group will encourage the use of specialized colleagues for help in diagnosis or treatment. Group practice will give the patient the advantages of access to a wider array of skills and facilities whenever they are needed."

And so the commission created a new medical specialty, replete with its own residency training program, to fill the void left by the now-moribund GP. The report recommended that in order to give comprehensive care, the primary physician should be schooled in internal medicine, psychiatry, pediatrics, medical gynecology and preventive medicine. Included in his or her graduate training should be "some experience in the handling of emergency cases and knowledge of the specialized care required before and following surgery."

Moving beyond the problem of the vanishing general practitioner, the Millis Commission recommended ways of improving residency training for all specialists. The members of the commission gave a strong vote of confidence to the basic soundness of the residency system but felt it needed lots of fine tuning. "Any basically sound system may, however, have troubles, and this one has its share," the report said. "The hospitals that offer residencies differ widely in quality, size, opportunity for diverse and progressive responsibility, and in commitment to educational objectives. In some teaching hospitals too few of the attending physicians are interested in teaching. In some there is little if any full-time staff. In some the resident's educational experiences and practice are poorly supervised and coordinated. In others the senior staff members are too involved in research to have adequate time for treating patients or for teaching residents. Many hospitals have difficulty in finding patients adequate in number and variety who can be assigned to the residents as their responsibilities."

Many of the commission's recommendations reflect Dr. Cole's ideas of how residency training should be set up. "For example, a period of fundamental training in general surgery (two to four years) before branching into the specialized surgical areas is advisable," the report states, "and a basic period of perhaps two years in medicine would advantageously precede branching into the medical specialties." The report went on to say one of the advantages of this basic training is that there would be "less compartmentalization of patients of particular types, greater flexibility in their use, and thus opportunities for broader and more varied experience on the part of each beginning resident."

At about the same time that the Millis Commission's report came out, Medicare and Medicaid appeared on the American scene for the first time. These government programs to finance medical care for the elderly and the poor were to have an enormous impact on every aspect of medicine, not the least of which was graduate medical education. In a speech before the 1967 Congress on Medical Education, sponsored by the AMA, Dr. Leland McKittrick from the Harvard Medical School reviewed the provisions of the Millis Commission report and had this to say about government's emerging role:

"The new role of government in assuming financial responsibility for all patients 65 and over and for all others unable to pay for their own care now places a responsibility upon it, not only in the payment of the hospital and resident staff but also in the quality of the hospital and medical care which these patients receive. The economic aspects of our programs in graduate education are not just academic. The increasingly heavy responsibility of third parties, especially government, in the care of patients on teaching services places those who are paying in a position to greatly influence the effectiveness of these programs. The importance of this must be recognized and faced in our future planning."

Government involvement—some in medicine would say intervention—rapidly became a major force in medical education and practice in the years following the Millis Commission report. Nonetheless, many of the Millis Commission's recommendations are now reality. The "primary physician" that the commission's report defined is variously called a family practitioner or primary-care physician today, and his or her role is crucial in an era of health maintenance organizations, preferred provider organizations and the pervasive group practice mode of medical care. Before the commission met, "the general practitioner was almost a disgrace to medical treatment. People were mad at him for making mistakes," Dr. Cole said in 1989. "As a result of the commission's recommendations, the general practitioner is now at a high level in terms of his ability."

Dr. Cole considered his appointment to the Millis Commission one of the highest honors his colleagues, ever paid him. In 1966, the American Medical Association gave Cole its Distinguished Service Award in recognition of his work for the association and for medicine in general. When John Millis sent Cole a copy of the commission's report, he wrote on the inside front page, "Dear Warren: With this personal copy of our report comes my warm personal gratitude for your great contributions. Now you will have to number me among those who have learned at your feet."

Dr. Cole's influence as a teacher was not only professional but personal as well. His former residents felt so personally attached to him that they formed the Warren H. Cole Society in 1959 to honor Dr. Cole and promote medical education. Originally formed by the 72 residents that Cole trained in general surgery, the society holds annual scientific meetings and sponsors a scholarship for an undergraduate medical student. Dr. Loring Helfrich became the first president of the society. When Dr. Cole retired in 1966, the Cole Society endowed the Warren H. Cole Professorship of Surgery at the University of Illinois.

Cole was clearly moved by this tribute. "Perhaps the most important personal item in my career as head of the department was the formation of the Warren H. Cole Society by my residents, close professional associates and research fellows in 1959," he wrote for the *Scope* in 1981. "This turned out to be perhaps the greatest honor I had ever received.

"The originators of the society were frank in saying that their respect and appreciation of the training they had received from me prompted them to form the society, which was designated also as an alumni organization. In addition, the founders requested President David Henry to designate the head of the department as the Warren H. Cole Professor."

The publication of the Millis Commission report in 1966 marked the end of Dr. Cole's career as professor and head of the department of surgery at the University of Illinois but not the end of his influence on medicine and surgery. Although he retired the same year, he wrote scientific articles and published books in his retirement years, he remained on editorial boards for medical journals and he lectured often on scientific topics.

Cole's surgical textbooks were widely used in medical schools. He collaborated with Dr. Robert Elman on five editions of their *Textbook of General Surgery*, from 1936 to 1952, then published a *Textbook of Surgery* under his own name in 1959. In 1963 and 1970, he collaborated with Dr. Robert M. Zollinger on the *Cole and Zollinger Textbook of Surgery*. According to Dr. C. Rollins Hanlon, former head of the American College of Surgeons, "His highly respected *Textbook of*

General Surgery, with Robert Elman as co-author, went through several editions and consolidated a reputation for clinical surgery that brought under his influence a host of aspiring surgeons from this country and abroad."

Cole was a pioneer in the science of surgery. In a way, the task of the Millis Commission represented the fulfillment of the promise of the rise of scientific medicine and surgery. The volume of medical research that followed the reforms in medical education that Flexner instigated led to an explosion in medical knowledge and the need to break that knowledge down into discrete medical specialties. Left in the lurch were general practitioners with outmoded training.

Cole's role in reforming medical education in the 1960s was certainly a significant and lasting one. But perhaps his greatest contribution was in the quality of surgical education he gave to a long list of surgical trainees over the 30 years he spent as head of the department of surgery at the University of Illinois College of Medicine. The Cole Society is an enduring tribute to that contribution.

CHAPTER 18

෯

WORLD RECOGNITION
AND RETIREMENT

Many of the young surgeons from the British Isles who went through Dr. Cole's residency training program as research fellows returned to their homelands and rose to prominence in their own right. In fact, several of his research fellows later became presidents of the Royal College of Surgeons of England or Edinburgh.

As Cole's influence spread, so did his reputation, not only in the United States but overseas as well. Through his research, teaching and published books and articles, he became widely known for his scientific accomplishments. In one year alone, 1959, he was made an honorary fellow of the both the Royal Colleges of Surgeons of England and of Edinburgh. In surgical circles, this is a high honor indeed. The Royal College in England limits the number of honorary fellowships they bestow to 100 living surgeons worldwide.

It was a triumphal trip that Warren Cole took to England and Scotland in July of 1958. His first stop was London where, on July 10th, he was admitted as an honorary fellow of the Royal College of Surgeons of England, an official body, first chartered by Queen Victoria in 1843, that issues certificates of advanced training in surgery. Professor Ian Aird from the Postgraduate Medical School of London, University of London, introduced Dr. Cole to the College's ruling council in this way:

"Warren Henry Cole has long been a friend of England and a personal friend of the members of this College. There are few of us here who have not experienced the warm hospitality of Dr. Cole and his charming lady in their delightful lakeside home in Chicago. Yet it is not on grounds of gratitude primarily that I present Dr. Cole to you now. He himself would, I think, like to be regarded in the first place as a research worker. In the case of some research workers, it takes lengthy descriptions to describe their productions, and sometimes the value of a piece of research is in inverse proportion to the space which must be devoted to describing it. Dr. Cole has made my task easy, for he has been responsible for important discoveries which can be described in a word.

"All of us in some measure hanker after immortality. Dr. Cole achieved that happy state 34 years ago when he was a young resident of 25 years of age. With Dr. Evarts Graham, he discovered cholecystography and thereby armed us all with one of the most important diagnostic weapons of modern times, and he opened a field which made possible the precise estimation of liver efficiency, which before him had not been possible. I find it a matter of regret that much of the colorful romance of his discovery has been destroyed subsequently by the chemists, and the rich purple liquid which we used to pour at dead of night into the veins of patients has been replaced now by a couple of tablets.

"In the later '20s and the '30s, Dr. Cole made other discoveries, important in surgery and pathology, which any of us would have been proud to make and which were secondary in importance only to his first achievement. In that time also he established himself, as not all surgical research workers do, as an operating surgeon of the first brilliance. For his operative field, he chose the tiger country of the hilum of the liver, and his cautious but single-minded and courageous advance in the vascular jungle towards the stump of a common duct stamps him as a surgeon not only of wisdom and carefulness but of courageous tenacity. In many other fields, and notably in respect of cancer of the thyroid gland, Dr. Cole made valuable contributions to surgical science in the years between the wars.

"It is fortunate that he got his surgical chair early, for he has built in the University of Illinois a teaching school and a research department second to none in the world. This has come to fruition in the post-war years, and in his later researches Dr. Cole has guided a brilliant young team straight to the heart of the cancer problem. Under his guidance, a sure method has been elaborated of detecting malignant cells in the venous blood leaving a tumor at operation and in the peripheral circulating blood, and he has inspired an all-American attempt to reduce by chemotherapy at and after operation the distant metastases which so often circumvent the cancer surgeon's work."

At the same time that Dr. Cole received this honorary fellowship, another American surgeon was awarded the same honor—Charles William Mayo, son and nephew of the famous Mayo brothers who founded the clinic that bears their name in Rochester, Minnesota. Both Mayo brothers had also been made honorary fellows of England's Royal College of Surgeons, one in 1913, the other in 1921. Charles Mayo became head of the clinic when his father and uncle died within three months of one another in 1939.

From London, Cole went to Edinburgh to garner his second honorary fellowship on July 15. This time he was introduced by W. Arthur Mackey, professor of surgery at the University of Glasgow Faculty of Medicine, who said in part:

"When I knew Warren Cole first in 1932, when he was associate professor of surgery at Washington University Medical School in St. Louis, my heart and mind were captured by this quiet, kindly, studious, industrious, intelligent, drily humorous man, spending most of his time in the laboratory and having, as it seemed to me, unreasonably little clinical responsibility compared with his juniors, the resident staff who carried out the greater part of the operating on the professorial unit.

"I was not fully familiar then with the principles far less the merits of the Halsted system of surgical training, with its three phases like those in the life history of that order of smaller living things [butterflies] that constantly delight and astonish us more cumbrous creatures with their energy, efficiency and beauty. Cole was then, as it were, pupating, completing his intellectual and technical development, and when he burst forth in 1936 to assume the professorship of surgery at the University of Illinois, what a magnificent imago he showed himself to be. Little can be added now to his splendor, but we are fortunate here to dispose an honor rarely conferred, and then only on the most distinguished."

It was another 21 years until he was inducted into the Royal College of Surgeons in Ireland as an honorary fellow in 1978, 12 years after he retired, but his scientific writing and activities in medical associations kept him in the forefront of medicine. His Irish sponsor to the Royal College of Surgeons made note of Cole's many medical involvements with characteristic Irish humor:

"Sir, in requesting that you confer the honorary fellowship of the College on this famous man, were I simply to recite his distinguished deeds, we should all have gravitational edema. Thus he is a member of 31 societies and associations and has been president of 15 of them. There are an additional 22 societies and associations of which he is a member, but fortunately for his bank balance, of these he is an honorary member.

"He has been president of the American College of Surgeons and an honorary fellow of the Royal College of Surgeons of England and also of Edinburgh. In Belfast in 1954, he was the Sir Thomas Dixon Lecturer and now, 25 years later, he has returned to repeat that performance and this time he also graces us by traveling to Dublin.

"And so, Mr. President, knowing that you yourself will be acquainted with his seven books and many of the 350 scientific articles, I will not bore you with a recitation."

Actually, the speaker underestimated the number of books that bear Dr. Cole's name as author or editor—his personal bibliography lists 13.

In addition to his honorary fellowships and 15 presidencies in various organizations, Cole was given a long list of awards throughout his career and even into retirement. Among them are:

- The Leonard Research Prize for the development of cholecystography (1926).
- The Distinguished Service Award from the University of

Kansas (1949).

- A National Divisional Award from the American Cancer Society (1953).
- The Roswell Park Medal, awarded by the Buffalo Surgical Society (1953).
- The Distinguished Service Award from Washington University (1955).
- The Modern Medicine Award for Distinguished Achievements (1956).
- The Gold Medal Award from the Radiological Society of North America (1960).
- The Distinguished Service Award from the Illinois Interprofessional Council (1962).
- The Distinguished Service Award from the American Geriatrics Society (1962).
- The Distinguished Service Award from the Cancer Prevention Center of Chicago (1962).
- The Chicagoan of the Year in Medicine Award (1964).
- The Senior Citizens Hall of Fame, Chicago (1965).
- The Distinguished Service Award from the American Medical Association (1966).
- The Edwin S. Hamilton Interstate Teaching Award from the Illinois State Medical Society (1966).
- An honorary Doctor of Science degree from Washington University (1967).
- The National Award from the American Cancer Society (1967).
- The Lucy Worthem James Award from the James Ewing Society (1969).
- The Edward Henderson Award from the American Geriatrics Society (1970).
- An honorary Doctor of Science degree from the University of Illinois (1970).

National and international recognition is one thing, but one of Dr. Cole's greatest personal honors came on the home front at the time of his retirement in June 1966. More than 500 guests gathered at McCormick Place in Chicago for a testimonial dinner for him on June 8. The dinner capped a two-day event planned by the Cole Society that included the reading of scientific papers by residents and colleagues.

On June 7, his surgical residents presented papers and attended a luncheon that featured Dr. Granville A. Bennett, dean of the College of Medicine, as speaker. After lunch, the residents went on grand rounds with Dr. Cole.

During the day on June 8, a list of heavyweights in surgery came to Chicago from around the country to give another round of scientific papers in honor of Dr. Cole. The speakers included Dr. Frank Glenn, then professor and head of the department of surgery at Cornell University in New York; Dr. R. Lee Clark, director of the M. D. Anderson Hospital and Tumor Institute in Houston; Dr. H. William Scott, Jr., professor and head of the department of surgery at Vanderbilt University in Nashville; and Dr. William P. Longmire, Jr., professor and head of the department of surgery at the University of California, Los Angeles. Dr. Joseph S. Begando, vice-president of the U. of I. at the medical center, gave a luncheon address.

On June 4, the Saturday before the testimonial, the *Chicago Daily News* published an article, written by science editor Art Snider, recalling Dr. Cole's life and career. Snider had written to Cole's former residents, friends and colleagues to solicit stories and anecdotes for the article. "At 68," Snider wrote, "Cole is an unlikely candidate for the rocking chair. He has the tanned, fit look of an outdoorsman. His hair, though thin, is still brown. The spring in his step is pronounced. The Izaak Walton look is no accident. He has spent countless hours with a fishing rod."

Snider quoted Dr. Ormand Julian, head of surgery at Presbyterian-St. Luke's Hospital, on Cole's passion for fishing. "Every July he sets up camp on the gravel bar on the Current River in Missouri and devotes himself to a series of eight- or nine-hour fishing days. His line handling with the fly rod shows the same dexterity that he displays in the operating room."

The fishing trips often included philosophic discussions around the campfire, Dr. Leon Bromberg, Cole's roommate for eight years in St. Louis, told Snider. "I recall Dr. Walter Alvarez lying in the hammock reading French poetry, Jim McDonnell (builder of the Mercury and Gemini spacecrafts) predicting for us things which then sounded like science fiction, and always the quiet and authoritative observations of Cole on subjects in or out of medicine."

Bromberg also recounted a time in the 1920s when Cole had a fondness for the evolving technology of aviation and spent many hours at Lambert Field in St. Louis where he became a friend of Charles "Slim" Lindbergh. Bromberg and Cole joshed Lindbergh about losing planes while he parachuted to safety, to which Lindbergh replied, "You can kid me all you want to, but after I win that $25,000 Orteig prize (for the first non-stop flight to Europe), I am going to be fixed for life."

Snider called Cole "an authority on the colon, stomach, gallbladder and thyroid. He is a specialist in cancer surgery and has developed a widely-copied method for drug prevention of cancer cell spreading after surgery. His surgery in the west side medical center is largely devoted to charity cases. Of these patients, he has frequently said: 'They have been put in my hands. The private patients can get a surgeon of their choice.'"

Dr. Hushang Javid, who served under Cole for 22 years as a student, intern, resident and faculty member, told Snider: "To me, the remarkable thing is that Dr. Cole, with his gentle, mild manner, plain appearance and a face that seldom shows an emotion, has left such a warm and endearing impression in the minds and hearts of the men he has trained."

One reason, Snider wrote, is that Cole sought to advance the careers of "his people" at every opportunity. A case in point was a story related by Dr. James H. Mason, who had responded to Cole's request to find a case history to illustrate a point for a book chapter the chief was writing. "He subsequently listed me co-author of the chapter," Mason said.

Another former resident, Dr. Robert G. Canham of Decatur, Illinois, said that the residents' affection for Cole "is like that of a son for a father."

More tributes came the following Wednesday night at Cole's black-tie testimonial dinner at cavernous McCormick Place. The main speaker for the evening was Cole's life-long friend, Dr. Alton Ochsner, who at that time was emeritus professor of surgery at Tulane University. Among the 500 present for the affair was the president of the University of

Illinois, David Dodds Henry, and most of the members of the university's board of trustees. Dr. Loring Helfrich, one of Cole's residents from 1940 to 1943, served as master of ceremonies.

Dr. Ochsner talked about the role of the physician in national and international affairs. "I think we physicians have been derelict in thinking that our only objective is to take care of patients," he said. "There's no question that is our primary objective, but we also have another objective—we have to be good citizens. And that role is best exemplified in Warren Cole's life. No one could have been a better citizen nationally or internationally than Warren Cole has been. I've known Warren ever since 1918 when he was a shy country boy. He was the child prodigy of our class. He was the youngest man in our class and the smartest. This man typifies everything that is right in medicine."

Dr. William Grove, a professor of surgery at Illinois and then the president of the Cole Society, presented a check to the president of the university to establish the Warren H. Cole Professorship of Surgery. When he accepted the check, president David Henry said, "I am happy to say to you, Dr. Cole, that the University of Illinois is a more distinguished and a greater institution because of what you have done. This is true in the lives of the countless patients you have served and the physicians you have trained.

"This gift places store on the values for which Dr. Cole has stood, the values that you have come to honor tonight. First is the desire to improve one's profession and the persistence he has shown in fulfilling that desire. The second is professional conduct of the highest order. And the third is personal and intellectual integrity. When these three attributes are put together as a pattern of values, they add a new dimension to the achievements upon which they rest."

Dr. Cole had his turn at the microphone to thank those present and to reflect on his life and career. "I'd like to tell all of you here that I am very grateful for the opportunity that I have had at the University of Illinois during the past 30 years. That has been my extreme good fortune. As a matter of fact, I have been lucky all of my life. I was lucky when I was accepted as a medical student at Washington University, because that allowed me to come into contact with Dr. Evarts Graham, who was the most inspiring man I ever met. Then I was lucky that in Dr. Graham's pyramidal system of residency, I was not dropped by the wayside after the first year.

"I'll also admit I was lucky when the animal caretaker failed to feed one of the dogs to which I had given tetra-iodophenolphthalein. I was lucky that I happened to read an article by the famous physiologist, Dr. Boyden of Minneapolis, who had just shown that food had a physiologic effect on the gallbladder of a cat. I had to know that before I could piece together the parts of cholecystography. We had to be able, for example, to appreciate the role of starvation in the success of cholecystogram. Then I was very lucky when I was offered the chair of surgery at the University of Illinois.

"But my luckiest day was when Clara Cole consented to join hands with me in walking down life's trail. The majority of my accomplishments since that date are due to her understanding, intelligence and her tolerance of my working night and day."

Cole officially retired on September 1, 1966, when Dr. Lloyd M. Nyhus succeeded him as chairman of the department of surgery and became the first Warren H. Cole Professor of Surgery at the University of Illinois. A 1947 graduate of the Medical College of Alabama in Birmingham, Nyhus had his residency training at the King County Hospital in Seattle under Dr. Henry N. Harkins and rose through the academic ranks at the University of Washington School of Medicine to become professor of surgery in 1964.

True to his nature, Dr. Cole applied a scientific method to his selection of a retirement locale. At age 68, he and Clara moved to Asheville, North Carolina, to a comfortable home on West Kensington Road overlooking Beaver Lake. He chose Asheville because it met a set of about 15 criteria he established for the ideal place in which to retire.

At the top of the list was climate. "But you have to be careful with that," he told a reporter for the Asheville *Citizen-Times*. "The average temperature can trick you. There was one place in California that had a mean temperature pretty close to that of Asheville. But its high temperature hit 115 degrees for three months of the year. Wouldn't want to live there at all. And there was one place in the Northwest that appeared to meet the climate test so far as temperature was concerned. But along with the other data I got from the chamber of commerce, there was the statement that 'Our city enjoys sunlight 104 days a year.' Now that figures out so that two out of every three days are overcast and probably rainy. That wasn't for us."

Also high on Cole's list of criteria was a requirement that his new home town be within 50 miles of an active trout stream. "And that really limited the field, let me tell you," he said. So all roads led to the city of Asheville, nestled in the Blue Ridge Mountains.

Although he found a place to retire, Cole went back to work. He continued writing scientific articles, he was active on the lecture circuit, and he published four books for which he was either editor or co-editor. He continued to serve on boards and commissions, and he attended national and international meetings on surgery and cancer. His schedule might have done in a younger man. It almost killed him in 1966, the same year he moved to Asheville.

He was returning from Buenos Aires where he had conducted a five-day seminar on cancer surgery with four other physicians. The lecture schedule was grueling, and his social commitments kept him up until 3:00 in the morning every night. On his return flight from New York to Roanoke, Virginia, he suffered a heart attack caused by coronary occlusion. He was unconscious when the plane landed in Roanoke. Fortunately, his wife and his doctor were there to meet him because they had planned a fishing trip together. He was rushed to the University of Virginia where he remained for about six weeks.

"I think that heart attack was a warning, part of the safety mechanism that God put into my body, into all our bodies, to warn us when we are pushing too hard," Cole said in 1978. "I still do things, but I pay some attention to my pulse rate. If the rate starts to rise while I'm working in the garden, for instance, I stop what I'm doing and do something else less vigorous."

With that cautionary attitude, Cole lived and worked in Asheville for 24 years, until 1990 when he died at the age of

91. He continued writing until his eyesight weakened, continued lecturing until he could no longer travel safely and continued fishing almost to the end.

Section Four:

⁊

The Retirement Years

Chapter 19

ॐ

Essays from Asheville

I n addition to his scientific writing, during his retirement years Dr. Cole also wrote essays full of personal remembrances about his life. Some are amusing, some touching, but all reveal aspects of the man's thoughts and personality.

In late 1985, he began a series of "Stories and Anecdotes by Dr. Warren H. Cole" which were never published but survived in his personal papers in typewritten form. Some of these stories have been quoted elsewhere in this book. What follows is a representative sampling of those essays.

HOW TO MAKE MONEY, THE SLOW BUT SAFE WAY

It is somewhat absurd to have a busy physician make remarks on how to get rich. My father was a poor farmer, and had told me what little he knew about economy. After World War I, we (the soldiers) were offered life insurance at a low cost. My father had life insurance but insisted that the insurance companies made a lot of money on their clients. He even suggested I drop my insurance—but take it up later if and when I got married. I did drop the insurance policy, and I was glad I did because it was this small accumulation of funds which allowed me to enter the stock market. My profits in the stock market made many times the "profit" on life insurance. I must confess that the funds which we have accumulated beyond a very modest amount are due entirely to my efforts in the stock market, namely six or seven securities purchased 50 or more years ago.

One of my very early investments was Chicago Flexible Shaft, recommended to me by my good friend Dr. Joseph Gale, who trained with me under Dr. Graham, and went later to Madison, Wisconsin, on the staff of the medical school. I had adopted strict prerequisites regarding purchase of securities. First, the company must have been making money and paying dividends for the past nine or ten years. Second, it must not be loaded with loans. The product must appear practical, but it is true that some of the companies with the most spectacular gains were making something new, e.g., computers and copy machines. Besides Chicago Flexible Shaft, I purchased National Dairy (later Kraft), Walgreen, Standard Brands, Lambert Chemical and International Harvester. I purchased these and put them away, hoping they would pay good dividends and split many times. All except one did; three were spectacular. The one which failed was International Harvester. However, it split once after my purchase, thus lessening the loss since I sold it before it went into bankruptcy. I also purchased some utility stock to stabilize the list; when a good utility company begins to lose, all it has to do is raise the rate.

I realize I was lucky. I do not recommend that everybody play the stock market.

HOW TO MAKE MONEY,
THE ACCIDENTAL BUT SAFE WAY

The tips in this category are of a different origin. They are usually very reliable but not commonly encountered.

One day in about 1928, I was talking with Dr. Graham and Dr. Malvern Clopton, a pediatric surgeon on Dr. Graham's staff. He was a fine surgeon, an excellent gentleman and a man with great integrity. Their conversation shifted, accidentally, I would say, to the stock market or, perhaps more accurately, to securities. I truly believe that Dr. Clopton did this intentionally. He knew that Dr. Graham had a very meager salary, and had no outside source of funds. He was actually recommending Lambert Chemical to Dr. Graham as a money maker, and hoping (I believe) that he would buy some. I don't know whether or not Dr. Graham bought any, but I did a few days later. Shortly after this, Warner Chemical bought Lambert Chemical, adopting the name Warner Lambert thereafter. The president of Warner Lambert was such a shrewd man that he caused his company to split many times.

Another "sure" tip I encountered was obtained in 1953 on a plane from New York to Chicago. Just before take-off a "young" man of about 55 years of age sat down next to me. He was a very pleasant fellow. We talked about many things that revealed our professional attachments. Before landing in Chicago he asked, "I suppose you are interested in making money?"

I replied, "Yes, but I don't have time to watch the stock market."

He continued, "If you were going to make a sure investment, how much money would you invest?"

I replied, "No more than $2,500. That would be all the money I could afford to lose." This apparently satisfied his thoughts lest I splurge with millions.

Then he surprised me. "I shouldn't do this, but I am glad to help out a professional man like you. I am a director of the X Company" (the name must remain unknown because he was breaking a rule) "and we just had a directors' meeting in New York. Our company is making money, and has been for the past several years. We voted to split six weeks from now and raise the dividends. If you invest in this, you must do so in the next few days because this news will leak out and the stock will rise sharply."

I had no reason to think he was talking wildly, so in a couple days I scraped up $2,650, the amount needed to buy 100 shares of their company. So, it apparently pays well to be friendly at all times. I am quite sure if Mr. X had not thought well of me, he would never have revealed the fact that his company was going to split in a few weeks. It split two or three more times in the next 10 years.

A VERY NARROW ESCAPE FROM DEATH

Dr. J. Albert Key, an orthopedic surgeon on the Washington University Medical School staff, and I were good friends; both of us loved fishing and hunting. We had been invited by Dr. Howard Naffziger and one of his orthopedic friends to go steelhead fishing on the Umpqua River in southern Oregon. As I recall, the steelhead "run" occurred on the Umpqua River early in September, just ahead of the opening of medical school. We would stay in a motel fishing resort—and did so every September for five or six years.

One year, when the steelhead fishing was poor, Albert and I asked the owner of the motel if there was a place near-by where we could do some trout fishing. He said, yes, there was a place where Calf Creek entered the Umpqua about a half mile above our camp. His directions were poor, but he assumed we would readily find it because the creek entered the river. The Umpqua was a fairly large river with a fast current and clear water. Strangely, the surface was smooth in spots of the fast current, thus confusing the wader, making him unaware of the danger of being swept downstream and hitting his head against the many rocks in the white water.

Dr. Key and I walked the bank upstream, and started across the river at a point which we thought corresponded to the point suggested by the owner. Actually, it was shallow except for the last 15 feet where the depth appeared to be four feet or slightly more. We started at this narrow stretch of deep water, knowing that the swift current would make crossing hazardous. We were using a wading stick, as was customary for wading the stream. This stick made wading in the shallow water much safer, but we knew a fast current could sweep one downstream in a hurry. Dr. Key was 40 to 45 pounds heavier than I was. We knew wading was much more dangerous for lightweight people.

Finally, Dr. Key said, "I can make it, so brace yourself while I go across." He started across. We were both amazed how strongly the current pressed him downstream. His feet were sliding downstream at a fast pace. His acceleration downstream increased. It looked bad.

I said to myself, "I'm going to lose one of my best friends, and I can't do a thing about it." Suddenly he stepped into a hole in the bottom, and the upper rim of his shoulder wader slipped under water. This allowed several gallons of water to fill his waders. This put more weight on the bottom and I saw the next few steps allow him to move toward the shore and grab a limb of a bush growing on the edge of the bank. He was able to crawl onto the bank just a few feet ahead of the white water and rocks.

When he got to his feet on the bank he let out a few cuss words and said, "That was much worse than I thought. I was lucky to get across." He told me I could never get across because I was 40 pounds under his weight.

I told him, "Maybe I can if you can find a long narrow pole, or cut one." He found one and began cutting it. The few minutes required for this seemed hours because I was now getting tired bracing myself while waiting. He finally cut it down and rushed to the bank opposite me. He cast the narrow end of the pole toward me, holding on to the other end. The tip fell short of my waiting hand by eight or ten inches and the fast current swept the pole so rapidly downstream that it was almost swept from his hand.

We both exclaimed, "That won't work!" I added, "I'm getting tired, but will go back to the other shore while you find someone who knows where the crossing is safe." While I was resting, he found three men, one of whom knew where the shallow water stretched all the way across. The safe crossing was only a hundred yards upstream. The three of them formed a chain, holding onto each other's hands so that if one slipped and fell the other would hold him. Using that system they crossed readily. I joined them and we returned safely. That was the closest call I had ever had.

MY PHYSICIAN IN ASHEVILLE

I have been fortunate in having Dr. Irby Stephens as my physician from the time of my coronary occlusion in 1966 to 1982 or '83 when Dr. Stephens retired. As a matter of fact, Dr. Stephens was at our house waiting for us to return from my air trip from Charlottesville, Va., where I spent about a month after having my heart attack on my way to Roanoke, Va. Mrs. Cole and I have been very favorably impressed by Dr. Stephens' willingness to leave his office to come to our home and examine me for any complications which I might have experienced from my air trip from Charlottesville.

Dr. Stephens graduated from Columbia University College of Physicians and Surgeons in New York in 1948. He spent two years (internship) at Columbia. At this point his training was interrupted by the war. When he returned from the war, he was invited by Dr. Longcope to come to Hopkins for his residency in internal medicine, where he stayed for four years. Dr. Longcope invited him to stay on in academic medicine there at Hopkins, but he declined.

When I asked him just recently why he chose to come to Asheville instead of staying in Baltimore, he replied, "My wife and I are from Arkansas, and I was not sure that I would fit into the academic life of Baltimore." Modest as always.

I had not had much contact with Dr. Stephens before I recognized he was a very capable and knowledgeable internist. My opinion was made indelibly so when I asked him a question about the cause of my coronary occlusion. My physician in Charlottesville had told me that I had very young arteries and he was very surprised to find that I had a coronary occlusion. It is true that I had been under considerable stress for a week before I had my occlusion. I had been attending a cancer meeting in Buenos Aires, Argentina, where I (with five or six other speakers) would come to the meeting at 8:30 a.m., stay all day, and go to dinner every night Monday through Friday. Going to dinner meant showing up at the host's address at 10:45 p.m., and having a drink or two before dinner was served about 1:45 a.m. We got to our hotel about 3:45 a.m., not getting over four hours of sleep. This was the schedule every day. I asked Dr. Stephens if this stress could have anything to do with my occlusion.

He replied, "Well, your surgical friends (quoting one or two) have shown that serious stress would shorten the clotting time of animals and human beings, just as hemorrhage would." This knowledge of another specialty amazed me. It showed that he was a widely read individual. Further contact with Dr. Stephens (as the years went by) confirmed this "well read" feature of his medical life. Very shortly I realized that Dr. Stephens was just as knowledgeable and capable in diagnostic medicine as any internist I had ever met. Only one internist in Chicago could match his skill and ability.

It was always a great treat to come to Dr. Stephens' office for my annual checkup because he would usually put me last on his list, so that there was no hurry to complete my examination to make room for another patient. This would allow us to spend as much as an hour (his willingness) to talk over various features of medicine. I have always felt very indebted to Dr. Stephens for his splendid medical care, and his willingness to spend extra time with me, talking over medical problems in general. He is an exceptionally capable internist in diagnosis and therapy.

HOW TO LOSE A GOOD FRIEND

There are thousands of ways to lose a friend. I would like to tell you about an unusual circumstance by which I lost one, or think I did.

Dr. Howard Naffziger was a very distinguished neurosurgeon who was professor and head of the department of neurosurgery at the University of California in San Francisco. I think he was also professor and head of the department of surgery for a period of a few years, but this point is not very pertinent to my story.

One day, I believe in 1949 or 1950, I received a letter from Dr. Howard Naffziger. Early in my surgical career I had become goods friends with Dr. Naffziger; I do not recall just how this friendship started, but our friendship was very sincere. I considered him a very valuable friend. He was a fine gentleman and a splendid neurosurgeon. I recall that he had nominated me to be the Secretary of the Committee on Surgery appointed by the Surgeon General early in 1942 to advise him on surgical problems occurring during World War II. He said (in his letter) that, speaking for the University of California, he was inviting me to spend six months as acting head of the department of surgery there in San Francisco. He gave no reason for suggesting this transfer. Of course, visiting professors are common, except that this period of six months—possibly four months—was an unusually long period.

I was not sure that my dean would look favorably on such a long period. I would, of course, have to find someone in my department who could and would take my place as acting head of my department during my term at California.

This was obviously a very splendid compliment.

Such a "term of office" would obviously interrupt all my Chicago activities. Although I had done this for three months for the State Department in 1948, that term was different— almost a command performance. Several weeks previously, I had agreed to accept a speaking engagement at the Pan Pacific Surgical Association meeting in Hawaii during the dates suggested. The Pan Pacific engagement would consume about an entire week. This would interfere so much with my California engagement that I would have to cancel the Pan Pacific engagement.

I wondered if this invitation to California might be a prelude to a formal invitation to become head of the department at California. If so and I turned it down, it would be very incongruous for me to accept this "visiting professorship" and not accept the California professorship. I was really happy at Illinois and I doubted very much that I would want to change from Illinois to California.

This reminded me very much of an incident occurring in St. Louis 20 or 30 years previously, when Dr. Graham told me that Johns Hopkins had invited him to be head of the department of surgery in Baltimore. At that time the head of the department of surgery at Hopkins was considered a very prestigious position, as of course it is now. Dr. Graham told me he had turned it down because it would interrupt many clinical series, which constituted material for his professorship. He mentioned his series of patients having resections of the lung for cancer as an example, saying there were many more almost of equal importance. He convinced me that this transfer would create a situation which would jeopardize his importance as head of the Hopkins department of surgery. This situation with Dr. Graham was an important circumstance which ultimately led me to turn down the California invitation.

I didn't realize that my turn-down of the California invitation would be taken so seriously by Dr. Naffziger, but he never again revealed the sincere friendly attitude which existed between us previously.

I found out later that he (Dr. Naffziger) found someone to be visiting professor, and a very distinguished surgeon (who was head of an important department of surgery) but for a period much shorter than originally presented to me.

THE ONLY SURE WAY TO MAKE MONEY
ON THE HORSES

The late Dr. Leon Bromberg was a long-time friend. This friendship began during our days of residency in Barnes Hospital in St. Louis (1921-1926). He loved sports—of all kinds. We were in St. Louis at that time. There was dog racing there, but no horse racing. In about 1927 or 1928 he accepted a medical job in Chicago.

One day he sent me a telegram saying, "Think about Sunbeam in the seventh." I had difficulty getting the correct meaning, but realizing that the word "seventh" actually meant the seventh race in one of the two or three race tracks in Chicago, I looked in the *St. Louis Post-Dispatch* for the results of the seventh race in Chicago. Sure enough, a day or two later Sunbeam was in that race—and he won. I didn't think much about this because anyone might get lucky and win one horse race.

To my surprise in five or six days I got another telegram saying, "Look up Lucky Day in the fifth." Again I looked in the *Post-Dispatch* the next day and, sure enough, Lucky Day won. This amount of luck could not happen to any one—the chances were one in a million. So I deduced he knew something about the races in Chicago.

So I became convinced that if I received another telegram I would bet. I scraped up $50, put it away and waited. No telegram arrived in five days. Two or three weeks later I got another similar telegram telling me to remember Starbeam in the fourth. I placed the bet after I found a reliable booker and waited; that horse "also ran."

The next day I wrote him a scorching letter. In a day or two I got a reply explaining the bad result. Dr. Bromberg was working two or three half-days per week in a charity clinic and had a black man as a patient who was improving physically under Dr. Bromberg's care. Two or three weeks before he sent me a telegram he told me that his patient (known as Lightning) asked him if he would like to make some money. Dr. Bromberg replied, "Sure. Everybody likes to make money."

Lightning said he was working as a stable man out at the race track and had accidentally overhead the jockeys fixing a race. He hid at that spot each day and discovered that every five or six days they fixed a race so the jockeys could bet and be sure to win. Lightning said that the races moved to another track, and he could not find where the jockeys were fixing the races. He said a couple weeks went by and, knowing that his doctor friend was waiting for more tips, he sent the doctor one of his own, but that horse did not win.

ADVANTAGES OF A LITTLE CULINARY KNOWLEDGE

As related elsewhere, I lost my mother at the age of four, and although my father hired housekeepers, there were many occasions when we had no such help. I was willing to accept the responsibility of cooking for the family, and my father agreed.

It was years after I actually cooked for the family (circa 1928) when four doctors including myself decided to go trout fishing in northern Wisconsin. Bill Gnagi of Monroe, Wisconsin, was one of the gang, and we were leaving from his home. The wives of two of the fellows bought the food and had it assembled in several boxes which we loaded into the car in which we were going to drive to the fishing camp.

My friend Bill Gnagi, who was two years behind me in Dr. Graham's training program, had made the arrangements to rent a cottage near the stream we were going to fish. Our cottage was near Crandon, Wisconsin, but Bill insisted we had to go to Argonne first. I argued with him, trying to get him to forget it and save time because I was a bit tired for the 300-mile drive. He insisted—saying it was only 15 or 20 miles extra and he had to pick up something very important to the fishing trip. Anyway, I finally agreed; it seemed I had to.

We found the town of Argonne. He instructed the driver to go this way one mile, that way one mile, to a sort of a log cabin. We went into the place, which turned out to be a saloon. Bill walked up to the boss, whom he knew. The boss said, "I'm glad to see you again, Bill. What can I do for you?"

Bill replied, "About one jug."

The boss turned to one of his helpers and said, "Joe, go out and get one." Joe went out the door and disappeared into the woods; shortly he returned with a gallon jug under his arm, obviously moonshine whiskey. Bill gave the boss a dollar or two and we continued on our way to the cottage.

When we arrived at the cottage, we began unloading the boxes of food. Suddenly one of the fellows stopped in his tracks and dropped his box, exclaiming, "Good Lord, here we are all set for a fine fishing trip, with a lot of food, and no one to cook it." He asked Bill if he could cook.

"No," was the reply, and the same reply came from Charlie, the fourth man. He turned to me. I saw a fine opportunity. I knew the ladies would buy everything in cans and I noticed all boxes contained canned food. All you had to do was open the can and warm the contents.

So I said, "I can cook, but cooking is a hot job and there are a lot of other chores which must be taken care of."

One of the fellows exclaimed, "I can make coffee."

I added, "Fine, that's your job. But there are a lot of other things more important and time consuming." So I began the assignment of jobs. "Bill, you can sweep out and make the beds. Joe, you can carry in water, and wood for the stove. Charlie, you can wash the dishes," and so on with a few other duties, such as cleaning fish. We got along very well, and caught a few fish. I fried them after wrapping them in corn meal. Of course they tasted good. We didn't catch enough to become tired of them.

On our last day we were finishing our breakfast when Joe turned to Bill and said, "Bill, I just thought of something."

Bill replied, "Go ahead. I hope it is great discovery."

"Well, Bill, I just want to remind you that a slick guy from the city has bamboozled us into a contract, where he exchanged a tiny bit of culinary skill for hours of hard labor and we didn't have sense enough to catch on. He must have worn out three or four can openers." Whereupon all burst into loud laughter.

"Well," I said, "you will have to admit that all those companies putting up good canned food have some good cooks, don't they?" Anyway, everybody appeared to be happy and had a good time.

SOME FISHING STORIES FROM THE SENIARD CLUB

When I became too old to fish the rocky streams around here, it was logical that I should join a private fishing club where the fishing is done from a boat or a smooth grass-covered bank. It happened that my friend, General George Stewart, also had that idea and joined such a club called the Seniard Hunting and Fishing Club, named after the Seniard Creek, which had been dammed up to form a small lake 25 to 30 miles from Asheville.

After allowing several months to elapse since his election to the club, he engineered my election to the club. The water in the small lake remains cool enough in the daytime of summer to support trout. Although trout do spawn and grow up in the lake, they are not of sufficient number and size to meet our fishing needs. So we stocked the lake with trout of various size.

We had one hazard on the lake, namely snakes, especially the copperhead. We were anxious to destroy these snakes so we would not be bitten by them. I remember one day I almost stepped on one on the bank. I must have jumped five feet into the air in my effort to avoid it. One of our members, General Craig, loved to shoot them. He was an excellent shot and had a military carbine which was very destructive in his hands against most anything, including snakes. It was a powerful gun which would probably shoot two or three miles.

He nearly always brought that gun along when we went fishing. One day I saw a copperhead about three feet long lying on the bank. I yelled to my friend Charlie (Craig) to get his gun. Just before he arrived at the spot near me, the snake started across the lake; he must have been 40 yards from General Craig. He raised his gun, and pulled the trigger after using no more than one second to take aim. He must have hit the snake on his ventral side four or five inches from his head. I would swear on a stack of Bibles that I saw a portion of that snake four or five inches in length explode with a lot of water two or three feet into the air. One or two of the fellows looking on weren't so sure the bullet would cut the snake in two and force the smaller part into the air. But Charlie was convinced a bullet from that gun would do that. Anyway, that snake sank to the bottom of the lake and was seen no more.

Sir Charles Illingworth from Glasgow was head of the department of surgery at Glasgow University in Scotland for years. He has contributed much to surgery, and I have known him for years. He is a great fellow who has worked hard all his life, taking little time off from his work. However, he retired a few years ago, and has been traveling a bit. Two years ago he came to the United States to see his old friend Professor George Smith, who had been professor of surgery at St. Andrews College of Medicine in Scotland. Smith came to the U.S. three or four years ago (his wife was a native of the U.S.), obtaining the position as head of the department of surgery at the Veterans Hospital in Fayetteville, North Carolina.

While Illingworth was visiting his friend Smith, he asked if his old friend Warren Cole lived in North Carolina. Professor Smith replied, "Yes, in Asheville, 200 miles from Fayetteville."

Sir Charles said, "I'd better to go to Asheville and spend the day with him. He won't like me anymore if I don't come by to see him." Anyway, they called me, and we made arrangements to see Charles. They drove down one afternoon, arriving one morning early, after spending the night at a nearby town.

I wanted to spend the day doing the things Charles would prefer. So I asked him what we should do. "Would you like to drive down to Biltmore and see Biltmore Castle and the horses there which are very special?" He replied apologetically that he had seen too many castles at home and had seen many fines homes.

I gave him a couple more possibilities which he declined very apologetically. Next I said, "Would you like to go out to our private hunting and fishing club and see some deer and wild turkeys, as well as catch a fish or two?"

Apparently he was waiting for this suggestion because he immediately said, "Fine, that is exactly what I would like to do."

So Clara packed a lunch and out we went to our club 25 or 30 miles into the country. Our club is only a mile from civilization but is reachable only by a narrow rough road, almost requiring a vehicle with four-wheel drive.

Just as we arrived at the clubhouse, we saw 15 or 20 deer grazing on the grass in front of the cabin. They showed no fear of us and apparently waited around to be fed some corn, which we promptly did. Twenty or 30 minutes later a flock of wild turkey wandered across the grassy plot. Sir Charles was quite excited about this and exclaimed, "Are they what you call wild turkey?" We assured him they were. After inspection of our cottage and immediate environs, I suggested we go up to the lake (less than a half mile away) and catch a couple of fish.

We drove up to the lake and set up a line with a rooster tail spinner on it. Our visitor was really quite ignorant about fishing equipment but caught on to spin casting faster than I thought he would. After a few minutes of coaching, I asked him to "cast one out in front." Let me remind you that Sir Charles had never caught a fish, and in fact had never gone fishing in spite of the fact that some of the best trout streams in the world are in Scotland. The first two or three casts he made were not good, but I persisted, saying, "It takes a little time to learn."

Sure enough, shortly he made a good cast. I added a few coaching remarks—keep the rod tip down, start reeling a little faster, be ready to hit him when he strikes, keep reeling consistently. Sure enough, just as I hoped and expected, a fish hit his lure. I repeated, "Hit him," which he did, and he began to reel his fish in. When he got the fish near the boat, I reached out and netted it. The fish was 13 or 14 inches long.

I knew there would be a reaction, because he had come with me all the way out to the club to catch a fish and here it was. His face was blank for a second or two, then it burst into a broad smile with a sharp but not loud "Hurrah!" He was a very conservative fellow, and not subject to loud expressions of emotion. "But I think I should cast one more," he said, and he did. We then went down to the clubhouse and ate lunch. The amazing feature is that he lived next to the best trout streams in the world but had never gone fishing.

On another occasion, almost six years ago, Mr. Geoffrey Oates, a surgeon from Birmingham, England, wrote me saying he was attending a meeting in Atlanta for a week or two and could he come by with his wife and take in a day's fishing. Of course I said yes. They arrived, but during the night early in December. I had already made arrangements with General Stewart to take us out to our fishing club in his jeep. George said it snowed six inches at his place (Crowfield), but he could get to the club with his jeep. Mrs. Oates had never been fishing before, so I took her out in our snow-covered yard and gave her some lessons in casting with a spinning rod. She learned fast, so fast that in 15 minutes she had the rudiments of spin casting.

Ordinarily we would never think of going fishing after a snow storm of this magnitude, but I realized that Professor Oates was an ardent fisherman. When asked if they (husband and wife) would like to do something else, they replied, "Of course not. We came 4,000 miles to go fishing and that we must do." We drove to Crowfield and from there General Stewart took us out to the club. The closer we got to the club, the deeper the snow appeared to be. The temperature was only about 1 degree Fahrenheit below freezing, so actually we were not cold. We found enough snow shoes for everybody.

I put Mrs. Oates on the bank where trout fishing was usually good. The rest of us scattered along the bank. I stayed near Mrs. Oates to be sure she caught some fish. Actually, fishing was good. Mrs. Oates caught the first fish, and was the first to catch her limit of four. She was like a five-year-old lad going through his Christmas presents. Professor Oates had only three fish in his creel, but he said he had caught others but had turned them back, hoping he could land a big one to keep. I knew this was true, because I had seen him throw two or three fish back, but didn't want to dig further into that story because his wife could say, "I have four fish and you only have three." All of us had a good time. Professor Oates was especially impressed. When writing to me later he always refers to his wife as "that fisherwoman."

DR. LORING HELFRICH AND YOUNGSTERS HAD NEVER HAD A PET DEER

Dr. Loring Helfrich was one of the many members of the Cole Society who came to Asheville on my 88th birthday

(July 1986). While here, the transmission of his car broke down and he had to spend two or three extra days in Asheville waiting for parts to arrive from Chicago. That time waiting for the repair job on your car to be completed really becomes monotonous. I thought I would try to help. Knowing that Dr. Helfrich and his two boys, 12 and 15, were ardent fishermen, I suggested one day that we go out to our fishing club. They agreed heartily.

We went out the next morning. I thought we would look around the cabins and environs before going fishing. Shortly after we arrived, a flock of 15 or 20 wild turkeys wandered across the grassy plot in front of our cabin. But there were no deer to be seen anywhere. I felt very guilty because I had told the boys I would show them a lot of deer. We waited—none showed up. Suddenly I remembered that scattering some corn in front of the cabin often brought some out. So I very confidently said, "Alright, I'll call some deer for you." That remark resulted in a lot of laughter from all three because they considered I was joking since in their neighborhood (Sikeston, Mo.) deer are very shy. At the sight of man in their neighborhood, all deer run for their lives.

I saw a fine opportunity to have some fun while feeding our deer. So I said nothing about our habit of calling deer to our front yard by banging on utensils while scattering the corn. I went over to a large chest filled with corn, scooped up a small bucket full and walked over to our front yard. At the same time I handed a smashed gallon can to one of the boys and said, "Here, make a lot of noise on that can while I scatter the corn." This again resulted in a guffaw of laughter because they thought I was just trying to put on a show. The boy to whom I had given the gallon can was making no noise so I grabbed the can from his hands and started banging on it with a large stick. That resulted in more laughter and some hissing. They began asking, "Where are the deer?" I told them so many of the does were taking care of their fawns, they were slow about eating. I knew this was true but for a moment thought they might be able to call me a fake. I remembered that General Craig had named one of the deer Rachel. So I began to call "Rachel." More laughter. In desperation I said, "Give me five minutes more." Just as I said that, a doe poked her head out from bushes on the edge of the grassy flat. As she took a few steps toward us, a smaller deer showed up (perhaps last year's crop), but the doe began staring northward at the junction of the grassy flat with the woods. That was a strange reaction. I wondered to myself if she might have a fawn nearby and was trying to make it stay put. I didn't suggest this; they might say, "Let's go fishing."

Finally the doe with her young friend began to walk toward us. All three of the fellows stopped in their tracks. They were deeply impressed and said so. Those deer were a bit slow coming up to the corn, so I asked, "Would you like me to make her break into a run coming up here?" The fellows still thought the deer would not come toward us, but would run away. One of them said, "Yes, do that and we will get you the grand prize." I remembered that our deer loved to hear whistling. So I broke into the best whistling I could produce. Sure enough, it worked; the deer broke into a run. I quickly urged my friends to retreat to the cabin to give the deer a chance to come up for the corn. We sat down on the cabin porch and watched the deer eat their corn. Suddenly the big doe stopped eating and stared northward into the grassy flat. She stood completely still, even stopped chewing. Something was troubling her.

A few seconds later the older boy exclaimed, "Look out there!" pointing to the middle of the field. There were a few bushes along the grassy flat, somewhat obscuring our vision. But shortly we saw what was troubling mama deer. Two young spotted fawns were running toward us. The doe broke into a trot running toward the fawns. The fawns and mother deer soon met. The fawns separated, one on each side of the mother deer and began feeding.

Dr. Helfrich exclaimed, "Well, I'll be ———."

The boys suddenly became very serious. One of them said, "Dr. Cole, we want to apologize. You take all the marbles. Your plan was a great success. You are a master magician."

I replied, "Yes, I agree that we have had a good show. But that business of having a mother doe nurse two fawns right out in plain sight was not in my script. That's the first time I have ever seen that." We ate our lunch (which my wife had packed) and then went to the lake. All three of the Helfriches are skillful fishermen. In a short time all had their limit. Later we picked up Mrs. Helfrich at the hotel; then Clara and I took them to our club for dinner. They were much impressed with the location of our club on the 16th floor where we could look over the lights of the towns in all directions.

YOU MAY GO BROKE OR GET RICH ON OIL

A lot of people in this world have lost their fortune or gained one from oil. While I was doing public health work in Eldorado, Kansas, I saw an example right before my eyes.

I was coming out the door of the hotel after finishing dinner one evening, when an acquaintance of mine called me by name, asking if I felt lucky tonight. I didn't know how to answer, since I did not know what kind of luck he was referring to. I hesitated but answered, "Well, yes, but certainly not unlucky." I walked over to shake hands with him and asked, "May I inquire as to what kind of luck you are referring?"

"I'd like to explain to you," he replied, but added, "Can you go with me for an hour, and I'll explain." He started walking me over to his car. I consented to the ride and as we got in, he remarked, "I sure need someone with me tonight who is having one of the luckiest days of his life because it means a lot to me tonight. I am Mr. Cannon, you may already know that. I come from 100 miles west. My wife and I got interested in oil leases a short time ago and before we knew it we had acquired a lease for 200 acres on the edge of the Still Water Pool. A year or two ago, I began drilling on our lease. My wife and I have $70,000 in cash or equivalent plus a small mildly profitable business."

"Mr. Cannon," I asked, "May I inquire how deep you have to drill, and if you have to go through any rock?"

"No rock," he replied, "and we only have to go down 1,600 feet, costing between $10,000 and $12,000 per hole. I have drilled six dry holes and this is my seventh and last one. No more money."

I added, "I can certainly sympathize with your plight. Yes, I already have my fingers crossed."

"The big point is," my friend added, "that this morning

Joe (meaning his driller) was down 1,600 feet and he was about to enter the sand which might contain oil. He told me to come back early this evening and I'll have the answer for you." Mr. Cannon was getting nervous and sweat was beginning to leak from his brow. There was no joking about his feeling, and I could now understand the situation. Actually I was getting nervous myself. "My lease is only about a mile down the road." Then silence. I felt that he might be uttering a quiet prayer or trying to clear his mind a bit.

Just then an oil derrick appeared. He shook in his seat and sped up a bit but not too fast. Both of us were now quiet. He turned the corner into his leased land and just then we saw a human form standing with an oily handkerchief waving violently. "Look!" he exclaimed, "this is Joe waving, that means we're in." At that point he stopped the car, jumped out and dashed over to Joe. Sure enough, Joe was just as anxious to strike oil on this seventh and last hole as was Mr. Cannon, although it meant not a nickel to him.

Oil is a fine friend and a mean enemy which has taken the last dollar from many a man. But I had just witnessed a happy occasion of an oil strike just before financial disaster.

WOULD YOU LIKE TO GROW ORCHIDS?

A lot of people think they would like to grow orchids. Orchids are beautiful and it's nice to have a beautiful flower now and then, especially if you are a woman. Well, anyway, I got caught on that. When we came to Asheville, my wife decided it would be nice to have a greenhouse, and maybe grow some orchids. This sounded like a good idea because I would have a lot of spare time. I haven't yet (Feb. 1987) had more than an hour or two of spare time throughout the week.

If you have normal employment, you ordinarily do not want a large greenhouse—a lean-to is sufficient in size. Another point I found out unexpectedly was that the rules and results are much different in small and large greenhouses. One very important point—get a book describing how to raise orchids.

Most orchids do not like much sunshine, so you will have to get some sort of plastic shade to put over the top of your greenhouse, or attach blue plastic sheets (which absorb

50 to 60 percent light) to the inside of your glass. In the summer when you will probably remove your orchids outside, cymbidium orchids will do best in full sun. Since there is a variable amount of sunshine, you will have to watch your plants to detect too much light. This may show itself in several ways. The plant may become pale or may show black patches of gangrene.

Naturally the plants need water. Ordinarily watering once a week is sufficient. They will need more if in a small container. The amount of air circulation will also alter the amount of watering. For a lean-to greenhouse, nine by 12 by 10, a small fan on medium speed will be adequate air circulation. If you water the plants too much, the roots will get soggy and perhaps necrotic. Too much watering may encourage growth of fungus (mold). This can be treated, but since I believe I have never had a fungus infection, I do not know how to use the anti-fungal agents. It may and will take you several weeks to determine how much to water. If you are going into the orchid business seriously, you must learn how to feel the orchid mix, and adjust watering accordingly. If a plant has a soft spongy feel, it is usually not dry.

Orchids need to be fertilized—usually about once a month. Numerous agents (e.g., Peters) are suitable. Lately I have been using Peters 10-10-10 or 20-20-20. They claim you should use 10-30-10 if the plant is ready to flower. The tendency is to use too much fertilizer. Use no more than half a teaspoonful for a gallon of water. I am talking about the soluble crystalline fertilizer, not the kind you use in grass.

Now I have a confession. About my only excuse to insert a couple of pages on orchids herein is because two or three years ago I raised a record plant which put out eight spikes and 24 flowers. It was a gorgeous orchid, a Cattleya Canhamanna. If you should run across one and have a few loose dollars, I hope you will purchase it, hoping it will turn out to be a record bloomer. Solitary orchids do quite well—especially if you spray them with water quite frequently (e.g., once per day). Make sure they get a little sunshine in the winter inside your house, and put them under the shade of a tree in the summer.

My Canhamanna soon filled the container and I had to

break it and transplant it. Orchids don t like to be broken up. Do it as gently and atraumatically as you can. Each segment bloomed well (two or three spikes) the next year, but it doesn t look healthy. I m afraid I handled it too roughly.

Now an important word about asepsis. Orchids need pruning but do it aseptically. When you are moving from plant to plant, don t use the same scissors without sterilizing them with iodine or other effective agents. Better still, use razor blades and discard them after using one on each plant.

CHAPTER 20

爲

DEATH AND REMEMBRANCE

I n the early morning hours on Friday, May 25, 1990, Dr. Warren H. Cole died in his sleep, two months shy of his 92nd birthday.

The previous November, he and his wife Clara had moved from their home on Kensington Road to a retirement community known as Givens Estates near the Asheville airport. Although the community offered ready medical care when they needed it, Clara missed their home and was unhappy there. The day before his death, Warren purchased a new home for Clara with the help of his then personal physician and friend, Dr. Robert Moffatt. He was said to be in satisfactory health on that day.

A group of surgeons who were members of the Cole Society chartered a plane in Peoria, Illinois, and flew to Asheville for a memorial service held at the Grace Covenant Presbyterian Church on Tuesday, May 29.

Throughout his retirement years, with the exception of a heart attack in 1966, Dr. Cole remained in good health, although he became more feeble and his eyesight weakened as the years added up. His work kept him mentally alert.

Cole continued his work in cancer and edited two books on the subject after he retired. The first was published by Appleton-Century-Crofts in 1969 under the title *Cancer of the*

Digestive Tract, Clinical Management. Dr. Tilden Everson, with whom he had worked on studies of spontaneous regression of cancer, was his co-editor. The second, published in 1970, under the title *Chemotherapy of Cancer*, was a natural outgrowth of his interest in the use of chemotherapy to kill cancer cells shed after surgery. Cole wrote a chapter on adjuvant chemotherapy.

Also in 1970, Cole and Zollinger published the ninth and final edition of their textbook of general surgery, which Cole began in 1936 with Dr. Robert Elman as his co-editor. In 1972, he and Dr. Charles B. Puestow, clinical professor of surgery at the University of Illinois, published the seventh edition of *Emergency Care: Surgical and Medical*, a book they first published in 1942 under the title *First Aid, Diagnosis and Management* in response to the United States entering World War II.

From 1968 until 1972, Cole gave more than 81 invited lectures at medical schools and medical society meetings on topics ranging from gastric ulcer to dissemination of cancer. In an obituary published in the *Bulletin of the American College of Surgeons* in August 1990, Dr. C. Rollins Hanlon remembered a time in 1984 when the Cole Society sponsored a scientific symposium in Ireland. "During one such overseas venture in 1984, the group participated in the year-long bicentenary celebration of the Royal College of Surgeons in Ireland. A paper related to basic biology of cancer, recapitulating earlier work on cancer dissemination, was presented by Dr. Cole himself to a delightedly incredulous audience." Cole also wrote scientific articles about his major areas of interest—the spread of cancer and the treatment of accidental injuries.

Not surprisingly, his scientific approach to life extended to the process of aging. In 1971, he published an article in the *Bulletin of the New York Academy of Medicine* titled "Problems and Opportunities for the Aged." In it he wrote, "All aged persons are aware of numerous frailties which envelop them. Their decreased strength, decreased stability, slower reaction, stiffness, decreased intellectual capacity, impaired memory, hearing, and eyesight, and decreased physical reserve make them recognize that they have lost their youth. Unfortunately, this regression in so many functions often creates mental depression, which at times becomes serious.

"All our organs are subject to the wear and tear of life. Some regenerate, e.g., liver, thyroid, bone, skin, mucosa; others regenerate slowly or not at all, e.g., brain, kidney, adrenal, cardiac, and skeletal muscle. The liver is one of the best examples of an organ which can regenerate extensively unless damaged by alcohol or by disease. A major part of the wear and tear of life is due to decreased vascular supply, chronic disease process, and hormonal deficiencies. Many reports indicate that people do not lose their intellectual powers as they grow older, although they may function more slowly than before. An unknown author has beautifully expressed the meaningful qualities of the aged with the statement:

'Youth is not a time of life, it is a state of mind. It is a temper of the will, a quality of the imagination, a vigor of emotions. Nobody grows old merely by living a number of years. People grow old only by deserting their ideals.

'Years wrinkle the skin, but to give up enthusiasm wrinkles the soul. Worry, doubt, self-disgust, fear and despair, these are the long years that bow the heart and turn the greening spirit back to dust. Whether 60 or 16, there is in every being's heart the lure of wonder, the undaunted challenge of events, the unfailing childlike appetite of what next, and the joy of the game of living.

'We are as young as our self-confidence, as old as our fear, as young as our desire, as old as our despair.'"

In 1975, at age 77, Dr. Cole donated his memorabilia to the University of Illinois Library of the Health Sciences in Chicago, including his academic gowns, medals, plaques, pictures, books and correspondence, which went into a special collection.

When Cole made his donation to the library, Dr. William J. Grove, one of Cole's residents who became executive dean of the College of Medicine at the University of Illinois, commented about his former chief, "The outstanding characteristic of Dr. Cole was his loyalty to his residents and students. He almost never failed to meet his teaching commitments. He'd travel hundreds of miles to make Saturday rounds or his Wednesday clinic. Dr. Cole stimulated young surgeons to engage in research and devoted many, many hours to helping residents design their research projects."

The same year, Dr. G. Howard Glassford, another of Cole's residents, who later became director of medical affairs for Hinsdale Hospital in the Chicago suburb of Hinsdale, sculpted a bust of Dr. Cole and presented the bronze casting to the U. of I. Health Sciences Library. It remains today on display on the first floor of the library building.

In 1985, when Dr. Cole was 87 years old, the editors of the *Journal of Surgical Oncology* planned a special issue of the journal, or Festschrift, as such a tribute is called, to be dedicated to Cole and his contributions to cancer surgery. Included in the issue was an unsolicited paper that Dr. Cole had submitted to the journal without knowing that the special issue would be dedicated to him. His topic was "The Increase in Immunosuppression and Its Role in the Development of Malignant Lesions."

In the foreword to the issue (November 1985), Dr. Lloyd Nyhus, Cole's successor at the University of Illinois, noted, "Although many of us are reminded of his pioneering work with Dr. Evarts Graham in developing the test for visualizing the gallbladder, it will be in the field of cancer that his most memorable work will be found." Nyhus also mentioned Cole's continued work on cancer, even at his advanced age. "On July 24, 1985, Dr. Cole celebrated his 87th birthday. That same month he published an erudite statement in the *Annals of Surgery* entitled 'Need for Immunologic Stimulators During Immunosuppression Produced by Major Cancer Surgery.'"

When Cole was close to 90, he and his wife set up an educational and philanthropic foundation in their own names. The president of the foundation, Dr. C. Rollins Hanlon, noted in his obituary of Dr. Cole, "Thinking always of others, he and Mrs. Cole in 1987 established the Warren H. and Clara Cole Foundation to assist the work of the University of Illinois through annual support of its department of surgery, of the Cole Society, and of selected individuals in the early stages of a research career. These annual disbursements for causes to which he contributed so much by personal work and example were memorialized publicly by the university's president as a wholly appropriate act by this great university surgeon and humanitarian."

One of the speakers at Dr. Cole's memorial service in Asheville was Dr. Stuart S. Roberts, a Cole resident in the late 1950s and early 1960s who worked with him on pioneering research into the spread of cancer cells and who went on to become clinical professor of surgery at the University of Illinois College of Medicine in Peoria. Roberts remembered Cole with admiration and affection. "Dr. Warren H. Cole was a great man. He was a master surgeon, a great teacher and a renowned research scientist. He tied together his surgery, his teaching and his research in a manner that neglected none of them. If you were to describe his professional life in one word, that word would be excellence."

Dr. Roberts went on to say, "Over the years, Dr. Cole earned the type of reputation that leads others to call for him when they themselves need an operation. He was truly a surgeon's surgeon. Furthermore, it could be said that Dr. Cole's residents have been characterized as excellent surgeons, which was a great credit to Dr. Cole and to the University of Illinois. Dr. Cole was often asked how he was able to train such good surgeons. His modest answer was that he picked good men or good women to start with."

Roberts chose an anecdote from his residency days to illustrate the respect that Cole had in the medical community. "I treasure one story which beautifully shows the measure of the man. When I was a senior resident, I received a long distance call from Dr. Papanicolaou, the famous Dr. Pap of the Pap smear. Dr. Papanicolaou did not want to bother Dr. Cole, who was then president of the American Cancer Society, but Dr. Pap's niece had been admitted to a New York hospital with metastases from carcinoma of the breast. He wanted Dr. Cole's opinion on the best treatment. To make a long story short, after Dr. Pap and Dr. Cole talked on the phone (it was 2:00 p.m.), Dr. Cole left on a 6:00 p.m. plane for New York and consulted on Dr. Pap's niece that same evening."

Another speaker at the memorial service, Dr. Philip E. Donahue, who was then president of the Cole Society and chief of general surgery at Cook County Hospital in Chicago, said: "Dr. Cole inspired by example. He led a simple life, was unassuming and unpretentious, and was dedicated to the pursuit of knowledge and the health of his patients and professional family. Patient care, education and research consumed virtually all his energy throughout his professional life.

"If the ultimate worth of a person's effort can be judged by the conduct which it inspires, then the daily efforts of generations of surgeons all over the world will continue to give evidence of Dr. Cole's excellence. His example is a prescription for professional and personal success: Continue the traditions and principles to which his life was devoted—selfless effort and dedication to patient care."

Commented Dr. Olga Jonasson in an interview after his death, "I think Dr. Cole will be best remembered for his great dignity and his obvious competency and the fact that he clearly had a tremendous breadth of knowledge and experience. He was a figure whom everyone respected. He carried that off very well. He was a distinguished role model to whom very few could aspire. As students, we were in awe of Dr. Cole's authority, his dignity and his knowledge."

According to Sir Geoffrey Slaney, "Dr. Cole will certainly, in my judgment, be remembered among the American greats of the last half of this century. I think the influence he has had on surgery, not only through his department and the number of surgeons he has trained—look at the number of people from his department who got into influential places in American surgery—but also through his work with the American College of Surgeons, the American Cancer Society and the National Cancer Institute. They kept him on the editorial board of journals like the *Annals of Surgery* until he was well into his eighties, I think. The peer-reviewed journals don't do that unless the person's opinions are highly regarded."

Dr. Cole's was a life full of accomplishment, dedication and fulfillment. His memory will live on not only in the minds of those he trained and influenced but also by virtue of the treatments he devised and the knowledge he uncovered. Dr. Cole's legacy is a body of research work that delved into many of the modern plagues of man, but most notably cancer.

His career is a symbol and analogy for the ascent of scientific surgery and the advent of the surgeon-scientist. His single lifetime represents the span of surgical care that began with a crude and bloody death following a kitchen-table operation in rural Kansas and ended with laser surgery, miraculous organ transplants and the seeds of genetic engineering to combat disease. Cole personally contributed to this growing wealth of scientific knowledge throughout his career and trained hundreds more to carry on the tradition, a tradition born just before the turn of the century at the Johns Hopkins School of Medicine and developed in academic medical centers across the United States throughout this century.

Cole was a quiet, even reticent man whose sheer dedication to teaching and research spoke volumes both in physical tomes and in the clear voice of scientific revelation. Not lost in all of his discoveries were countless numbers of patients who have and will receive the direct therapeutic benefits of his analytical mind. His life and work surely place him, as Sir Geoffrey Slaney put it, among the greats of American surgery in the last half of the 20th century.

But perhaps among all the accolades, Warren Cole should have the last word in his biography. When asked to reflect on his chosen profession in 1959, he said, "I've had fun every day of my life...and how many people can say that about their jobs?"

BIBLIOGRAPHY

Chapter 1

Bonner, Thomas Neville: The Kansas Doctor, A Century of Pioneering. Lawrence: University of Kansas Press, 1959.

Glaser, Hugo: The Road to Modern Surgery, The Advances in Medicine and Surgery During the Past Hundred Years. New York: E.P. Dutton & Co., Inc., 1962.

Hertzler, Arthur E.: The Horse and Buggy Doctor. New York and London: Harper & Brothers, 1938.

King, Lester S.: American Medicine Comes of Age 1840-1920. Chicago: American Medical Association, 1984.

Ludmerer, Kenneth M.: Learning to Heal, The Development of American Medical Education. New York: Basic Books, Inc., 1985.

Morrison, Samuel Eliot: The Oxford History of the American People. Vol. 3, 1869-1963. New York and Scarborough, Ontario: New American Library, 1972.

Rosen, George: The Structure of American Medical Practice 1875-1941. Philadelphia: University of Pennsylvania Press, 1983.

Rothstein, William G.: American Physicians in the Nineteenth Century, From Sects to Science. Baltimore and London: The Johns Hopkins University Press, 1972.

Wangensteen, Owen H. and Sarah D.: The Rise of Surgery, From Empiric Craft to Scientific Discipline. Minneapolis: University of Minnesota Press, 1978.

Chapter 2

Boorstin, Daniel J.: The Americans, The National Experience. New York: Vintage Books, A Division of Random House, 1965.

Howard, Robert P.: Illinois, A History of the Prairie State. Grand Rapids, Michigan: William B. Erdmans Publishing Company, 1972.

Morrison, Samuel Eliot: The Oxford History of the American People. Vol. 3, 1869-1963. New York and Scarborough, Ontario: New American Library, 1972.

Streeter, Floyd Benjamin: The Kaw, The Heart of the Nation. New York and Toronto: Farrar & Rinehart, Inc., 1941.

Chapter 3

Britt, Albert: An America That Was, What Life Was Like on an Illinois Farm Seventy Years Ago. Barre, Massachusetts: Barre Publishers, 1964.

Boorstin, Daniel J.: The Americans: The Democratic Experience. New York: Vintage Books, A Division of Random House, 1974.

Croy, Homer: Corn Country. New York: Duell, Sloan & Pearce, 1947.

Foght, Harold Waldstein: The Rural Teacher and His Work. New York: The MacMillan Company, 1917.

Griffin, Clifford S.: The University of Kansas, A History. Lawrence: The University Press of Kansas, 1974.

Hamilton, Carl: In No Time At All. Ames, Iowa: The Iowa State University Press, 1974.

McGovern, George (ed.): Agricultural Thought in the Twentieth Century. Indianapolis and New York: The Bobbs-Merrill Company, Inc., 1967.

Chapter 4

Bonner, Thomas Neville: The Kansas Doctor, A Century of Pioneering. Lawrence: University of Kansas Press, 1959.

Beveridge, W.I.B.: Influenza: The Last Great Plague, An Unfinished Story of Discovery. New York: Prodist, A Division of Neale Watson Academic Publications, Inc., 1977.

Flexner, Abraham: Medical Education in the United States and Canada, A Report to the Carnegie Foundation for the Advancement of Teaching. New York: Arno Press & The New York Times, 1972.

Griffin, Clifford S.: The University of Kansas, A History. Lawrence: The University Press of Kansas, 1974.

Ludmerer, Kenneth M.: Learning to Heal, The Development of American Medical Education. New York: Basic Books, Inc., 1985.

Olch, Peter D.: Evarts A. Graham in World War I: The Empyema Commission and Service in the American Expeditionary Forces. Journal of the History of Medicine and Allied Sciences, vol. 44, no. 4, pp. 430-446, Oct. 1989.

Osborn, June E. (ed.): Influenza in America, 1918-1976. New York: Prodist, A Division of Neale Watson Academic Publications, Inc., 1977.

Chapter 5

Connaughton, Dennis: Alton Ochsner: Not As a Legend. Bulletin of the American.College of Surgeons, vol. 66, no. 5, May 1981.

DeCamp, Paul T.: Alton Ochsner (1896-1981). Journal of Cardiovascular Surgery, vol. 23, pp. 88-89, 1982.

Flexner, Abraham: Medical Education in the United States and Canada, A Report to the Carnegie Foundation for the Advancement of Teaching. New York: Arno Press & The New York Times, 1972.

King, Lester S.: American Medicine Comes of Age, 1840-1920. Chicago: American Medical Association, 1984.

Lippard, Vernon W.: A Half-Century of American Medical Education: 1920-1970. New York: Josiah Macy, Jr. Foundation, 1974.

Ludmerer, Kenneth M.: Learning to Heal, The Development of American Medical Education. New York: Basic Books, Inc., 1985.

Numbers, Ronald L.: The Education of American Physicians, Historical Essays. Berkeley, Los Angeles & London: University of California Press, 1980.

Olch, Peter D.: Evarts A. Graham in World War I: The Empyema Commission and Service in the American Expeditionary Forces. Journal of the History of Medicine and Allied Sciences, vol. 44, no. 4, pp. 430-446, Oct. 1989.

Rothstein, William G.: American Medical Schools and the Practice of Medicine. New York and Oxford: Oxford University Press, 1987.

Chapter 6

Carroll, Douglas: The Bayview Asylum: The Influence of a University (1891-1911). Maryland State Medical Journal, pp. 117-119, July 1966.

Carroll, Douglas: The Bayview Asylum: Clinical Medicine (1911-1934). Maryland State Medical Journal, pp. 69-71, Aug. 1966.

Cole, Warren H.: The Development of Cholecystography. Surgical Rounds, pp. 24-32, Mar. 1982.

Finney, J.M.T.: A Surgeon's Life. New York: G.P. Putnam's Sons, 1940.

Harvey, A. McGehee; Brieger, Gert H.; Abrams, Susan L.; and McKusick, Victor A.: A Model of Its Kind: A Centennial

History of Medicine at Johns Hopkins (Vol. I). Baltimore and London: The Johns Hopkins University Press, 1989.

Hawley, Paul R.: Medicine as a Social Instrument: The Hospital and the Community. New England Journal of Medicine, vol. 244, no. 7, pp. 256-259, 1951.

Supervisors of City Charities: 23rd Annual Report to the Mayor and City Council of Baltimore. City of Baltimore, Department of Charities and Correction, 1922.

Thomas Richard Boggs. Bulletin of the Johns Hopkins Hospital, vol. 63, pp. 349-350, 1938.

Turner, Thomas B.: Heritage of Excellence: The Johns Hopkins Medical Institutions, 1914-1947. Baltimore and London: The Johns Hopkins University Press, 1974.

Chapter 7

Brock, R. Lord: Evarts A. Graham. Annals of Thoracic Surgery, vol. 9, pp. 272-279, 1970.

Cole, Warren H.: Compensatory Lengthening of the Femur in Children After Fracture. Annals of Surgery, vol. 82, pp. 609-615, Oct. 1925.

Cole, Warren H.: Results of Treatment of Fractured Femurs in Children. Archives of Surgery, vol. 5, pp. 702-716, Nov. 1922.

Cole, Warren H.: Systemic Blastomycosis (Oidiomycosis). Annals of Surgery, vol. 80, pp. 124-134, 1924.

Coller, Frederick A.: The State of the Association. Annals of Surgery, vol. 120, p. 265, 1944.

Lippard, Vernon W.: A Half-Century of American Medical Education: 1920-1970. New York: Josiah Macy, Jr. Foundation, 1974.

Olch, Peter D.: Evarts A. Graham: Pivotal Figure in American Surgery. Perspectives in Biology and Medicine, vol. 26, no. 3, pp. 472-485, Spring 1983.

Olch, Peter D.: Evarts A. Graham, The American College of Surgeons, and The American Board of Surgery. Journal of the History of Medicine and Allied Sciences, vol. 27, no. 3, pp. 247-261, July 1972.

Rothstein, William G.: American Medical Schools and the Practice of Medicine. New York and Oxford: Oxford University Press, 1987.

Chapter 8

Bordley, James III and Harvey, A. McGehee: Two Centuries of American Medicine, 1776-1976. Philadelphia, London & Toronto: W.B. Saunders Company, 1976.

Cole, Warren H.: A Reminiscence: Cholecystography—Its Development and Status. Review of Surgery, vol. 20, no. 6, pp. 373-378, Nov.-Dec. 1963.

Cole, Warren H.: Historical Features of Cholecystography. Radiology, vol. 76, no. 3, pp. 354-375, Mar. 1961.

Cole, Warren H.: The Development of Cholecystography: The First Fifty Years. The American Journal of Surgery, vol. 136, pp. 541-560, Nov. 1978.

Cole, Warren H.: The Story of Cholecystography. American Journal of Surgery, vol. 99, pp. 206-222, Feb. 1960.

Chapter 9

Cole, Warren H.: Chronic Appendicitis. Journal of the Missouri State Medical Association, vol. 32, pp. 369-372, Sept. 1935.

Cole, Warren H.: Evarts Ambrose Graham, 1883-1957. Bulletin of the American College of Surgeons, vol. 42, p. 138+, 1957.

Cole, Warren H. and Womack, Nathan A.: Reaction of the Thyroid Gland to Infections in Other Parts of the Body. Journal of the American Medical Association, vol. 92, pp. 453-457, Feb. 9, 1929.

Cole, Warren H.: Retroperitoneal Hemorrhage Simulating Acute Peritonitis. Journal of the American Medical Association, vol. 96, no. 18, pp. 1472-1474, 1931.

Cole, Warren H.: The Role of Hepatic Insufficiency in Surgical Problems. Journal of the Missouri State Medical Association, vol. 30, no. 9, pp. 351-355, Sept. 1933.

Cole, Warren H.: Suture Wounds of the Heart. Annals of Surgery, Vol. 85, pp. 647-652, 1927.

Cole, Warren H. and Womack, Nathan A.: The Thyroid Gland in Infections. Journal of the American Medical Association, vol. 90, pp. 1274-1276, Apr. 21, 1928.

Davis, D. J.: Biennial Report to the President for the Years 1934-1936. Annual Report of the University of Illinois College of Medicine. Chicago: Special Collections, University of Illinois Health Sciences Library, 1936.

Hatfield, Philip M. and Wise Robert E.: Radiology of the Gallbladder and Bile Ducts. Baltimore: The Williams &

Wilkins Company, 1976.

Meade, Richard Hardaway: An Introduction to the History of General Surgery. Philadelphia, London, Toronto: W.B. Saunders Company, 1968.

Way, Lawrence W. and Pelligrini, Carlos A.: Surgery of the Gallbladder and Bile Ducts. Philadelphia, London, Toronto: W.B. Saunders Company, 1987.

Womack, Nathan A. and Cole, Warren H.: Effect of Caffeine on Basal Metabolism. Proceedings of the Society for Experimental Biology and Medicine, vol. 31, pp. 1248-1250, 1934.

Zeman, Robert K. and Burrell, Morton I.: Gallbladder and Bile Duct Imaging, A Clinical Radiologic Approach. New York, Edinburgh, London, Melbourne: Churchill Livingstone, 1987.

Chapter 10

Bonner, Thomas Neville: Medicine in Chicago, 1850-1950. Madison, Wisconsin: The American History Research Center, Inc., 1957.

Cole, Warren H.: Opportunities for Surgeons in Medical Research. Journal of the American Medical Association, vol. 116, pp. 2543-2545, May 31, 1944.

Cole, Warren H.: 30 Years: The Department of Surgery. The Scope, Special Centennial Issue, p. 32, 1981.

Cohen, Edward P. (ed): Medicine in Transition, The Centennial of the University of Illinois College of Medicine. Chicago: University of Illinois Press, 1981.

Davis, David J.: College of Medicine Report to the President for the Year 1941-1942. President's Papers, Special Collections, University of Illinois Health Sciences Library, Chicago.

Davis, Loyal: J. B. Murphy, Stormy Petrel of Surgery. New York: G. P. Putnam's Sons, Inc., 1938.

Kittle, C. Frederick: The Development of Academic Medicine in Chicago. Surgery, vol.62, no. 1, July 1967.

Kiefer, Joseph H.: Town and Gown in the '30s. The Scope, Special Centennial Issue, pp. 35-36, 1981.

Ludmerer, Kenneth M.: Learning to Heal, The Development of American Medical Education. New York: Basic Books, Inc., 1985.

Ricketts, Henry T.: Forty Years of Full-Time Medicine at the University of Chicago. Journal of the American Medical Association, vol. 208, no. 11, June 16, 1969.

Ward, Patricia Spain: A Medical Center is Born, 1925-1938. The Scope, Special Centennial Issue, pp. 17-19, 1981.

Ward, Patricia Spain: Ophthalmology at Illinois, A Retrospective of the Illinois Eye and Ear Infirmary and the Department of Ophthalmology of the University of Illinois College of Medicine. Brochure, University of Illinois at Chicago, 1985.

Chapter 11

Bordley, James III and Harvey, A. McGehee: Two Centuries of American Medicine, 1776-1976. Philadelphia, London & Toronto: W.B. Saunders Company, 1976.

Cole, Warren H.: Minutes of Committee on Surgery, National Research Council, Division of Medical Sciences acting for the Committee on Medical Research of the Office of Scientific Research and Development, October 23, 1943. Typed Report, Cole Papers, Special Collections, University of Illinois Health Sciences Library, Chicago.

Cole, Warren H. and Elman, Robert: Textbook of General Surgery. New York: D. Appleton-Century Company, Inc., 1948.

Cole, Warren H.: Differences Between Civilian and Military Surgery. Mississippi Valley Medical Journal, vol. 66, pp. 52-55, 1944.

Earle, A. Scott (ed.): Surgery in America, From the Colonial Era to the Twentieth Century. New York: Praeger Publishers, 1983.

Lada, John (ed.): Medical Statistics in World War II. Washington, D.C.: Office of the Surgeon General, Department of the Army, 1975.

NATO Handbook: Emergency War Surgery. Washington, D.C.: Government Printing Office, 1958.

Rankin, Fred W.: Letters to Warren Cole, March 19, 1942, and March 11, 1943. Cole Papers, Special Collections, University of Illinois Health Sciences Library, Chicago.

Wangensteen, Owen H. and Sarah D.: The Rise of Surgery, From Empiric Craft to Scientific Discipline. Minneapolis: University of Minnesota Press, 1978.

Chapter 12

Cole, W.H.: Carcinoma of the Colon. Rocky Mountain Medical Journal, vol. 42, pp. 169-178, 1945.

Cole, W.H.: Carcinoma of the Colon. Illinois Medical Journal, vol. 91, pp. 229-239, May, 1947.

Cole, Warren H.: Confidential Report on Present Conditions of

Surgery in Great Britain. Typed Report, Cole Papers, Special Collections, University of Illinois Health Sciences Library, Chicago.

Cole, Warren Henry: Operative Technic. New York: Appleton-Century-Crofts, 1949.

Cole, W.H. and Burch, G.E.: The National Health Service Act of England and Wales. American Practitioner, vol. 3, pp. 95-102, 1948.

Cole, Warren H. and Rossiter, Lewis J.: The Breast. Hagerstown, Maryland: W.F. Prior Co., Inc., 1944.

Cole, W.H. and Rossiter, L.J.: Chronic Cystic Mastitis: With Particular Reference to Classification. Annals of Surgery, vol. 119, pp. 573-590, 1944.

Cole W.H., Slaughter D.P. and Majarakis J.D.: Carcinoma of the Thyroid Gland. Surgery, Gynecology & Obstetrics, vol. 89, pp. 349-356, 1949.

Fraser, Derek: The Evolution of the British Welfare State. London: MacMillan Education Ltd., 1989.

Humphrey, Loren J.: Scientific Contributions of Warren H. Cole. Unpublished Paper.

Trail, Richard R.: The History of the Popular Medicine of England. Cambridge: Papworth Industries, 1965.

Chapter 13

Cole Committee: Statement by the Research Validation Committee, June 24, 1953. Typed Report, Cole Papers, Special Collections, University of Illinois Health Sciences Library, Chicago.

Goldman, Robert P.: The Fantastic Krebiozen Story. The Saturday Evening Post, vol. 237, pp. 15-19, Jan. 4, 1964.

Krebiozen Research Foundation: Krebiozen. Brochure, Special Collections, University of Illinois Health Sciences Library, Chicago.

Newspaper Files on Krebiozen. Special Collections, University of Illinois Health Sciences Library, Chicago.

Marbarger, John P.: Minutes of the General Faculty Meeting, November 19, 1952. Special Collections, University of Illinois Health Sciences Library, Chicago.

Stoddard, George D.: "Krebiozen": The Great Cancer Mystery. Boston: Beacon Press, 1955.

Stoddard, George D.: The Pursuit of Education: An Autobiography. New York: Vantage Press, 1981.

Ward, Patricia Spain: "Who Will Bell the Cat?" Andrew C. Ivy and Krebiozen. Bulletin of the History of Medicine, vol. 58, pp. 28-52, 1984.

Young, Warren R.: What Ever Happened to Dr. Ivy? Life, Vol. 57, pp. 110-126, Oct. 9, 1964.

Chapter 14

Balfour, Donald: Private letter to Warren H. Cole, December 18, 1954. Special Collections, University of Illinois Health Sciences Library, Chicago.

Bordley, James III and Harvey, A. McGehee: Two Centuries of American Medicine, 1776-1976. Philadelphia, London & Toronto: W.B. Saunders Company, 1976.

Cole, Warren H.: Measures to Combat the Menace of Cancer. The American Surgeon, vol. 17, no. 7, July 1951.

Cole, W.H.: Recurrence in Carcinoma of the Colon and Proximal Rectum Following Resection for Carcinoma. Archives of Surgery, vol. 65, pp. 264-270, 1952.

Cole, Warren H., Packard, Douglas and Southwick, Harry W.: Carcinoma of the Colon with Special Reference to Prevention of Recurrence. Journal of the American Medical Association, vol. 155, pp. 1549-1553, 1954.

Davis, Loyal: Fellowship of Surgeons, A History of the American College of Surgeons. Springfield, Ill.: Charles C Thomas, 1960.

McGrew, Elizabeth A., Laws, John F. and Cole, Warren H.: Free Malignant Cells in Relation to Recurrence of Carcinoma of the Colon. Journal of the American Medical Association, vol. 154, pp. 1251-1254, 1954.

Shimkin, Michael B.: Contrary to Nature. Washington, D.C.: U.S. Government Printing Office, 1977.

Wangensteen, Owen H. and Sarah D.: The Rise of Surgery, From Empiric Craft to Scientific Discipline. Minneapolis: University of Minnesota Press, 1978.

Chapter 15

Bordley, James III and Harvey, A. McGehee: Two Centuries of American Medicine, 1776-1976. Philadelphia, London & Toronto: W.B. Saunders Company, 1976.

Cole, Warren H. (ed.): Chemotherapy of Cancer. Philadelphia: Lea & Febiger, 1970.

Cole, Warren H.: Presidential Address, American Cancer Society, Inc., October 26, 1960. Unpublished typescript, Special Collections, University of Illinois Health Sciences Library

Chicago.

Cole, Warren H.: Spontaneous Regression of Cancer. CA, vol. 24, pp. 274-279, 1974.

Cole, Warren H.: Surgery and Ancillary Methods of Therapy for Cancer (Editorial). American Surgeon, vol. 25, pp. 986-987, Dec. 1959.

Cruz, Ernesto P., McDonald, Gerald O. and Cole, Warren H.: Prophylactic Treatment of Cancer. Surgery, vol. 40, pp. 291-296, 1956.

Everson, Tilden C. and Cole, Warren H.: Cancer of the Digestive Tract. New York: Meredith Corporation, Appleton-Century-Crofts, 1969.

Everson, Tilden C. and Cole, Warren H.: Spontaneous Regression of Cancer: Preliminary Report. Annals of Surgery, vol. 144, pp. 366-383, Sept. 1956.

Everson, Tilden C. and Cole, Warren H.: Spontaneous Regression of Cancer; A Study and Abstract of Reports in the World Medical Literature and of Personal Communications Concerning Spontaneous Regression of Malignant Disease. Philadelphia: W.B. Saunders Company, 1966.

Everson, Tilden C. and Cole, Warren H.: Spontaneous Regression of Malignant Disease (Guest Editorial). Journal of the American Medical Association, vol. 169, pp. 1758-1759, Apr. 11, 1959.

Morales, Francisco; Bell, Millar; McDonald, Gerald O.; and Cole, Warren H.: The Prophylactic Treatment of Cancer at the Time of Operation. Annals of Surgery, vol. 146, pp. 588-595, Oct. 1957.

Chapter 16

Cole, Warren H.: Annual Report of the Department of Surgery, July 6, 1949. Archives, University of Illinois Library, Urbana, Ill.

Cole, Warren H.: Annual Report of the Department of Surgery, June 21, 1950. Archives, University of Illinois Library, Urbana, Ill.

Cole, Warren H.: Mechanisms and Obligations in the Teaching of Trauma. American Journal of Surgery, vol. 93, pp. 493-497, Apr. 1957.

Cole, Warren H.: Surgical Philosophy Old and New, Address of the President. Bulletin of the American College of Surgeons, vol. 41, no. 2, pp. 67-71, Mar.-Apr. 1956.

Cole, Warren H. and Schneewind, John H.: The Teaching of Trauma at a University Hospital. Bulletin of the American College of Surgeons, vol. 40, pp. 204-206, Jan.-Feb. 1955.

Cole, Warren H.: 30 Years: The Department of Surgery. The Scope, Special Centennial Issue, p. 32, 1981.

Dowling, Harry F.: Building a department of medicine. The Scope, Special Centennial Issue, pp. 30-31, 1981.

Hering, Alexander C.: Traumatologia, Notes of a peripatetic trauma-watcher. Bulletin of the American College of Surgeons, vol. 63, no. 10, pp. 6-10, Oct. 1978.

Humphreys, James W., Jr.: General surgery redefined in the era of specialization. Bulletin of the American College of Surgeons, vol. 69, no. 7, pp. 4-6. July 1984.

Ludmerer, Kenneth M.: Learning to Heal, The Development of American Medical Education. New York: Basic Books, Inc., 1985.

Snow, James B., Jr.: The importance of general surgery to surgical specialists. Bulletin of the American College of Surgeons, vol. 69, no. 7, pp. 7-8, July 1984.

Ward, Patricia Spain: "Who Will Bell the Cat?" Andrew C. Ivy and Krebiozen. Bulletin of the History of Medicine, vol. 58, pp. 28-52, 1984.

Chapter 17

Citizens Commission on Graduate Medical Education: The Graduate Education of Physicians. Chicago: American Medical Association, 1966.

Cole, Warren H.: Annual Report, 1956-1957, Emergency Service, Research and Educational Hospitals, University of Illinois. Special Collections, University of Illinois Health Sciences Library, Chicago.

Cole, Warren H.: Mechanisms and Obligations in the Teaching of Trauma. American Journal of Surgery, vol. 93, pp.493-497, April 1957.

Cole, Warren H.: 30 Years: The Department of Surgery. The Scope, Special Centennial Issue, p. 32, 1981.

Hanlon, C. Rollins: Warren H. Cole, former College President, dies. Bulletin of the American College of Surgeons, vol. 75, no. 8 pp. 28-29, Aug. 1990.

McKittrick, Leland S.: Rational Responses to Graduate Education of Physicians. Journal of the American Medical Association, vol.

201, no. 2, pp. 112-114, July 10, 1967.

Schneewind, John H. and Cole, Warren H.: Emergency-Room Service in Hospitals. American Journal of Surgery, vol. 98, pp. 544-549, Oct. 1959.

Chapter 18

Aird, Ian: Admissions to the Honorary Fellowship. Annals of the Royal College of Surgeons of England, vol. 23, pp. 199-200, 1958.

Citation for Honorary Fellowship Conferred on Warren H. Cole. Archives, Royal College of Surgeons in Ireland, Dublin.

Henry, David Dodds: Acceptance for the University. Unpublished transcript, retirement party for Warren H. Cole, Special Collections, University of Illinois Health Sciences Library, Chicago, 1966.

Mackey, W. Arthur: Conferring of Honorary Fellowship on Dr. Warren H. Cole and Dr. I. S. Ravdin. Journal of the Royal College of Surgeons of Edinburgh, vol. 6, pp. 74-77, 1958-1959.

Moore, Bill: Dr. Warren H. Cole: Man of Many Honors. Asheville Citizen-Times, July 16, 1978.

Ochsner, Alton: The Role of the Physician in National and International Affairs. Unpublished transcript, retirement party for Warren H. Cole, Special Collections, University of Illinois Health Sciences Library, Chicago, 1966.

Over 500 Gather for Testimonial to Dr. Cole. University of Illinois Medical Center News, vol. 21, no. 8, p. 2, June 1966.

Snider, Arthur J.: An Honored Surgeon—And a Lovable Guy. Chicago Daily News, June 4, 1966.

Chapter 19

Cole, Warren H.: Stories and Anecdotes by Dr. Warren H. Cole. Unpublished Essays, Special Collections, University of Illinois Health Sciences Library, Chicago, 1985-1987.

Chapter 20

Cole, Warren H.: Problems and Opportunities for the Aged. Bulletin of the New York Academy of Medicine, vol. 47, no. 11, pp. 1318-1330, 1971.

Donahue, Philip E.: In Memory, Warren H. Cole, M.D. Unpublished typescript of memorial service for Warren H. Cole, Special Collections, University of Illinois Health Sciences Library, Chicago, 1990.

Hanlon, C. Rollins: Warren H. Cole, former College President, dies.

Bulletin of the American College of Surgeons, vol. 75, no. 8 pp. 28-29, Aug. 1990.

Nyhus, Lloyd M.: Warren H. Cole, MD, FACS, FRCS. Journal of Surgical Oncology, vol. 30, no. 3, p. iv, Nov. 1985.

Roberts, Stuart S.: Words of Remembrance. Unpublished typescript of memorial service for Warren H. Cole, Special Collections, University of Illinois Health Sciences Library, Chicago, 1990.

Warren H. Cole Donates Memorabilia to Library of Health Sciences. University of Illinois Medical Center News, May 1975.